Stretch

Also by Neal Pollack

The Neal Pollack Anthology of American Literature
Beneath the Axis of Evil
Never Mind the Pollacks
Chicago Noir (editor)
Alternadad

Stretch

The Unlikely Making of a Yoga Dude

Neal Pollack

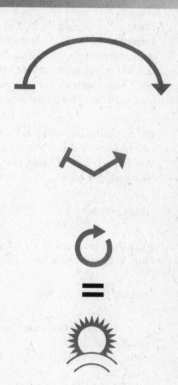

HARPER 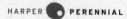 PERENNIAL

NEW YORK • LONDON • TORONTO • SYDNEY • NEW DELHI • AUCKLAND

HARPER ● PERENNIAL

HarperCollins books may be purchased for educational, business, or sales promotional use. For information, please write: Special Markets Department, HarperCollins Publishers, 10 East 53rd Street, New York, NY 10022.

FIRST EDITION

Portions of this book appeared, in slightly or substantially different form, in *Yoga Journal, Slate, The Faster Times,* and *Howl.*

Designed by Aline C. Pace

Library of Congress Cataloging-in-Publication Data
Pollack, Neal, 1970–
    Stretch: the unlikely making of a yoga dude/Neal Pollack.—1st ed.
      p. cm.
    ISBN 978-0-06-172769-6
1. Hatha yoga—Humor. 2. Exercise for men—Humor. I. Title.
RA781.7.P655 2010
613.7'046—dc22

                                              2010007873

10 11 12 13 14 /RRD 10 9 8 7 6 5 4 3 2 1

For Patty Pierce, Mara Hesed, and Richard Freeman,
most honored teachers.

"You are old, Father William," the young man said,
"And your hair has become very white;
And yet you incessantly stand on your head
Do you think, at your age, it is right?"

Lewis Carroll, *Alice's Adventures in Wonderland*

Contents

Acknowledgments

Doing yoga properly is straight up impossible without kula, or community, and I've been blessed with a wonderful kula of people throughout my practice and the writing of this book. I can't thank them enough, so a mention on the first page will have to do. We'll start with Regina and Elijah, my wife and son, whose support, love, and humor have given me ballast through some turbulent years; my parents Bernard and Susan Pollack; my sisters Margot Hummel and Rebecca Smith and their broods; Aunt Estelle and Uncle Larry; the King Brothers; the Dougherty cousins; Jon and Debbie Buxer; Uncle Rick and his imaginary farm; and the rest of my enormous family. Jerod and Joanne Gunsberg, Ben Brown, Katie Spence, Lauren Piscopo, and Bill Thomas have been true friends. Special thanks to Vanessa Grigoriadis, whose friendship and knowledge of the yoga world informed this book in many important ways, and to Beth Ann Fennelly, for reading early drafts and giving vital suggestions.

Also, many thanks to my teachers, Patty Pierce, Mara Hesed, and Richard Freeman, who pointed me down the right path, and other yoga teachers and friends who provided companionship, humor, guidance, and support along the way: Nina Mikkelsen, Julie and Eric Hunnicutt, Tanya Greve, Linda Richards/Prabhu Prakash, Liz Beckham, Robert Birnberg, Amber

Rothwell, Heather Funston, Hilary Kimblin, Deb Schoeneman, Catie Lazarus, Gregg Tolliver, Aubrey Hackman, Jennifer Presutti, Kelly Wood and all the sevas at Karuna Yoga, including Alex Cuesta, Laura Park, Ellen Monocrousoss, and Juliet Nussbaum. I'm also very grateful to Dhyana Justl and "Denise" (the only person in the entire book whose name I changed, and I'm still not sure why), my Canadian road-trip buddies, who gave me quite an adventure, and for my Thailand friends, especially Maria Türke but also Helmut and Gloria Bachmann, Karen Anderson, Cooper Schell, Marisa Hiltermann, Christiana Meissnitzer, and Romana and Sascha Delberg, along with the staff and faculty of Yoga Thailand, who run a tight ship, and the staff of the Easy Time, who run a loose one. From Wanderlust, special shout-outs go to Andy Langer and Kristine Pauls, Christy and Jason Marsden, Sandee Fenton, and Shelby Meade.

On the business end of my life, so to speak, many thanks to Diane Anderson and Dayna Macy at *Yoga Journal*, Josh Levin at Slate, and Sam Apple and Adam Baer at *The Faster Times*. At Harper, I'm grateful to David Hirshey, Amy Baker, and Carrie Kania for allowing me to come back to the fold, and to George Quraishi, for doing all the work. Also thanks to Daniel Greenberg, Shawn Simon, Shari Smiley, and Tiffany Ward for agenting and managing my silly career.

As for the famous yoga teachers who I (gently) mock in these pages, well, that's what I do, but all respect to their practice and to their incalculable contributions to yoga in the West. If I've forgotten anyone else, I sincerely apologize, but I want to keep this kind of short. Until the next book, then, I'll say: Namaste, motherfuckers!

Neal Pollack
Los Angeles, California
March 2010

Introduction: How Did I Arrive at This Ridiculous Place?

Early one Monday afternoon in the fall of 2009, I balanced on my right foot in a yoga studio in the San Fernando Valley. I leaned my body forward, just barely touching down my right fingertips, opened my body toward the west wall, and lifted my other arm and leg to the sky. This was *artachandrasana*, half-moon pose. I had to apply all my effort and concentration to get there, which wasn't easy because I was busy checking out the 40 other people in the room, none of whom I knew, and none of whom, I guessed, I would have liked if I had. They just looked so L.A. This wasn't my usual spot to practice, but I'd found myself in the neighborhood with a free hour and a yoga mat in the trunk of my car, and the $5 "lunchtime flow" class fit my tight budget.

I executed a technically sound Warrior Three, leaning forward on one foot while shooting my arms toward the front of the room in a vague imitation of Superman. Then I reached back, grabbed my outstretched foot with one hand, arched my chest, and extended upward. This was called bow pose, and again, I could get there if I tried. This involved activating my *bandhas*, focusing on my breath, ignoring the crappy Eric Clapton song that was playing, and realizing that the rooting down of my leg and the rising of my arm was all part of the same system, the magical alchemy of opposites that, when properly applied, helps me to understand the mysteries of the universe while sweating like a hog in the tropics.

Below, my natural rubber mat had begun to feel a little squishy. Though I wore a silky sleeveless tank top and comfortable stretchy shorts, it didn't prevent the sweat from flowing off me until I felt like Paul Newman in *Cool Hand Luke* after he'd spent that night in the box. My Dodger-blue sweat-absorbent mat cover with a grippy bottom and a soft, slip-resistant top, a much-loved birthday present from my wife, didn't really help, given the extreme volume of my *schvitz*. The bright orange circular *drishdi* at the top of the mat cover had nearly vanished because I'd washed it so often. It no longer provided a reliable gazing point.

I patted my neck, forehead, and armpits with my Manduka-brand hand towel, which I received in a swag-bag of freebies at a recent yoga festival, and crouched into child's pose. The instructor, who looked frighteningly like Jennifer Aniston, cleared her throat, ready to deliver some wisdom. I snorted some salty water up my nose and raised my head.

"So did everybody have an awesome Halloween weekend?" she asked.

Seriously? I thought, and then answered to myself: *No, not really. I took my kid trick-or-treating, ate a couple of peanut-butter cups, and went to bed early, like I do every night, because I can't afford a goddamn babysitter.*

The teacher's weekend, on the other hand, had been

quite awesome: A bunch of people had come over for a dinner party, and everyone was so good-looking and smart, and they made her feel really nice about herself because they were such amazing friends. Now I officially hated her. If you take a five-dollar class, you get a five-dollar teacher.

"So just remember, guys, to be grateful for everything you have," she said. "And after we do some more poses, I'll tell you about my costume."

How did I arrive at this ridiculous place? Five years previous, when my exercise routine had deteriorated to a half-hour on the elliptical followed by two or three beers, it was inconceivable. The men I knew didn't do yoga. We watched basketball and drank beer, played video games and guitar (or at least video games *about* playing guitar), quoted lines from cartoons, got stoned continually, and held all-night poker tournaments. Yes, I read books and my Netflix queue was full of foreign films, but that just put me on the more intellectual edge of the Dude Nation spectrum. Yoga didn't occur to me, ever. Why would it have? EA Sports, which comprised most of my interaction with matters athletic, never put out a yoga game.

But now, yoga had become my major hobby, my only non-work activity that didn't involve high-grade medical marijuana or baseball statistics. If I went more than twenty-four hours without yoga, my hips started to hurt. I sat in half-lotus while watching Sunday Night Football. Instead of eating hoagies, my previous life's noontime activity, I took lunchtime flow classes in the Valley.

After fifteen minutes of side planks, high lunges, crescents, twisted triangles, and bent forward half-lotuses, all of which left my skin as slick as a Sunday bookie, the instructor delivered on her promise.

"On Halloween, I dressed like Alice in Wonderland," she said.

I admit the thought of this loathsome woman wearing a powder-blue pinafore caused a little stirring in my loins. But thanks to my extremely sophisticated yoga training, I was able to observe this sensation and let it go. She continued:

"And a bunch of friends and I went to West Hollywood for the Halloween parade. It was a totally great scene. Everyone was really drunk. Some guy actually came over and looked up my dress. Isn't that offensive?"

The other students in the class, a predictable mix of Sherman Oaks housewives and gay men, expressed shock in the form of gasps and tongue clucking. They were obviously regulars. *Snap snap snap*, went their metaphorical fingers.

"There were like so many people in Lady Gaga costumes," the teacher said.

"Oh my God!" exclaimed the guy next to me. "I *love* Lady Gaga!"

Excuse me, I thought. *Aren't we supposed to be doing yoga here?*

"I'm not sure about her," said the teacher. "I think she's kind of a slut."

"She is *not* a slut," said the fan boy.

The room began to cluck. Everyone had an opinion. *Stop it, people*, I thought. *This is exactly what Lady Gaga wants you to be talking about! Don't you see that you're falling into her trap?*

But they didn't see, and I couldn't make them. I could only control myself, and my reactions to their unbelievably stupid conversation. So I took a small sip of water, pushed back into downward dog, and waited for the room to quiet down. Yoga, after all, is the art of self-mastery, of stilling the mind's—not to mention the mouth's—endless yammering, of the search for a peace beyond thoughts and words. The world was full of morons, and many of them did yoga from time to time, but that wouldn't stop me from practicing. Nothing would, anymore.

Stretch

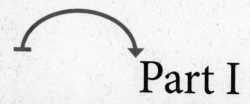

Part I

Find a Comfortable Seat

Yet Another Doughy, 35ish White Man

In the summer of my sixteenth year, I attended Anytown USA, a weeklong camp in the mountains of Northern Arizona. Since 1952, Anytown has intended, according to its website, "to bring together diverse youth from disparate backgrounds and overcome isolation, segregation, and discrimination, and to work toward the realization of democracy." A bit ambitious, perhaps, but it's a surprisingly successful ongoing project. Every summer, hundreds of Arizona "teen leaders" head up north and return a week later determined to fight bigotry in all its forms.

Most of the kids at Anytown weren't white, which wouldn't have been a big deal for someone who'd grown up in, say, Brooklyn, but it made for a very different kind of experience for a kid from suburban Phoenix in the 1980s. For the first time, I found myself feeling a common humanity with all different kinds of people, while also participating in three-hour long workshops on internalized racism. It all just felt so beautiful and perfect. I enjoyed it a hell of a lot more than Hebrew School. Every night, we sat around the campfire, surrounded by brooding pines. A counselor played the guitar and we sang the camp's theme song:

> *Anytown*
> *Anytown*
> *Yellow, black, white, red, or brown*
> *Makes no difference*
> *When you come down*
> *To Anytown*
> *Our Anytown*

We all linked arms, cried gentle tears of happiness, and confessed many wonderful things to one another. A big Native American kid named Dennis wrapped me in a monster hug and told me that he loved me like his brother and that we'd always be friends, even though he lived on the reservation and I lived in Paradise Valley, an exclusive suburb best known as the home of the Barry Goldwater Memorial. The only other time I ever saw him after camp was when his tribal dance troupe performed at an assembly at my high school. But at that moment, it didn't matter. I believed.

The real kicker, though, came on the camp's second-to-last day, when our counselors woke us at 4 AM and hustled us into the center of the compound. They divided us into groups and gave each group distinctly colored armbands. I was hoping I'd get put into a different group than usual, but nope, there I was again with the Jews. We were no longer, they told us, allowed to speak with anyone from another group. They didn't belong to the same camp, and they weren't our friends.

Take a group of smart, sensitive teenagers, strip them bare of their defenses, and then hit them where they're the weakest. That's a recipe for lifelong brand loyalty. The great social experiment lasted until about a half hour after breakfast, when the whitest, most privileged girl in camp tore off her armband, howled, "We're all the same inside!" and fell to the ground, sobbing. Much rending of armbands ensued, except for one of the Mexican guys, who refused to take off his band, and, I later heard, refused to talk to anyone but Mexicans for the rest of the summer.

I, on the other hand, returned from camp full of brightness, energy, and a desire to change the world. Suddenly, everyone was my friend. Back at school, I joined a club called H.U.G.S. The acronym stood for Human Understanding through Growth and Development, and the membership largely comprised former Anytowners. Who knew what the hell we did, but who cared? We had love.

There were other, more concrete manifestations of my joyous spirit. I volunteered at a soup kitchen and a homeless shelter. In a state that refused to acknowledge Martin Luther King Jr.'s birthday as a federal holiday, I took time out on that day to read Dr. King's "I Have A Dream" speech over the morning announcements. I'm sure plenty of people wanted to beat me up; they usually did. But for once, I didn't care. My mind, body, and soul were working in perfect unison. I was a young man transformed.

Ten years, countless manic-depressive episodes, and many failed relationships later, I found myself in my late twenties, working as a moderately successful and only slightly disillusioned weekly newspaper reporter in Chicago. I produced long, earnest stories that occasionally crusaded for social justice. In my experience, which didn't yet encompass Dick Cheney, Osama bin Laden, and many other villains of the George W. Bush era, Mayor Richard M. Daley was the most evil person on Earth.

But deep within my bowels, larger ambition brewed. I started writing little essays that made fun of contemporary journalism. They had titles like "This Albanian Life" and "Portrait of an Andalusian Horse Trainer," and they dripped with the same potent combination of aesthetic loathing and professional jealousy that has launched so many literary careers throughout the centuries. True to the late slacker era, I debuted them at an art gallery called Poop Studios, in the basement of Wicker Park's Flat Iron Arts Building. It had a little stage in the back. With the help of someone who I wanted to be my girlfriend, I built a scale model of a Chicago tavern, wrote a fake history of that tavern, and then destroyed it on stage with my Doc Martens. I was going to have trouble finding a wider audience.

Then, in what can only be described as the most astonishing break of my life, a friend of mine forwarded me an email from the writer Dave Eggers. He was starting a magazine called *McSweeney's,* and he was looking for contributions that the traditional glossies wouldn't touch. That pretty much described my work, so I sent the parodies to him, along with a variety of humor pieces making fun of Chicago politicians.

Unlike now, there was at the time little national interest in Chicago politics. On the other hand, essays satirizing obscure magazine pieces commanded the widest possible attention, and Eggers published them all as the lead piece in the first issue of *McSweeney's*, which is now a collector's item whose first autographed edition sells on eBay for hundreds of dollars. Another issue followed, and then a *McSweeney's* website. I wrote for both, and attended many parties. Soon, I began receiving email from random fans telling me how awesome and amazing I was and asking me when I would publish a book. They didn't have to wait long.

The Neal Pollack Anthology of American Literature came out in September 2000 after having been thought up the previous January. The "author" of the book, "Neal Pollack," was The Greatest Living American Writer, a seventy-something contemporary of Norman Mailer's and Gore Vidal's, more professionally accomplished and sexually experienced than the two of them combined. He was a parody, and an archetype, of American literary lionhood. At that point, though, no literary star shone brighter than The Dave's, and my book was the first one that he'd chosen to edit and publish himself. We got a four-page spread in *Men's Journal,* and a really positive review in the *New York Times,* which said that the book "works surprisingly well given its narrow premise." A gossip site called *My Manifesto,* dedicated to chronicling the culture surrounding *McSweeney's,* did a special post devoted my "rise."

The buzz bin overflowed.

A crazy book tour followed. I nearly got arrested for reading in the women's bathroom of the 30th Street Train Station in Philadelphia, staged a sandwich-eating contest at Zingermann's Delicatessen in Ann Arbor, hosted a weight-lifting demonstration at Venice's Muscle Beach, and performed at a discount Atlanta bookstore dressed as Mark Twain. A public radio intern followed my wife and I around on tour, recording parts of the adventure for a documentary. The attractive, nerdy, eager-to-please young people who came to my gigs by the dozens laughed and laughed as I gave thunderingly faux-pretentious authorial answers about the "decline of the American ego." Perhaps you had to have been there.

Suddenly, the world was predicting great things for The Nealster, as I used to call myself. In The Year Of Our Lord 2000, *Rolling Stone* named me its "Hot Writer." The following year, the now-defunct *Book Magazine* called me a "writer to watch," putting me on the cover alongside Jonathan Franzen and Jonathan Safran Foer, among others. At the time, when asked how this felt, I said, "I don't even own a watch. I hope they give me one." I thought I could afford to be flippant because *Entertainment Weekly* said I "looked great in fatigues." They knew this because the *Anthology* contained several shirtless portraits of me. The paperback edition went further, featuring an author photo where I lay naked on a white leather sofa, surrounded by books, typewriters, and bottles of booze, holding a frightened fluffy white cat in front of my crotch.

Soon, the Greatest Living American Writer had a column in *Vanity Fair* and I was opening for They Might

Be Giants at the Bowery Ballroom. Also, I appeared as a guest humorist on *Wait, Wait Don't Tell Me*. In my crowning moment, I read fake slam poetry in front of hundreds at the National Theater of Holland while David Byrne played percussion behind me. I'd always wanted to be a professional writer, and now I was having the time of my life, stumbling around drunk at a level many writers never reached, being treated as a near equal of the most celebrated young authors of my time. It felt exactly as I'd always imagined it would: glorious, except better. Also, people gave me free drugs, and I usually accepted them. The whole thing was just such a fucking miracle, like I'd gone to a winter fantasy workout and ended up cracking the Dodgers' starting rotation. So what if it was a bit of a gimmick, even a total sham?

Then, even more quickly than they'd arrived, the good times went away. One night somewhere in 2002, Eggers and I gave a reading at the Dallas Art Museum. He was charming and respectable. I sweated a lot because I'd eaten two pot brownies that I'd picked up at a book-tour stop in Madison, Wisconsin. While he read, I sat with my arms crossed, often snorting dismissively. At a party afterward, while I got even *more* stoned, Dave kindly came up to me, put a hand on my arm, and said "I want things to be more straightforward from now on."

From there, the dominoes fell quickly. The *Vanity Fair* column ended, and so did the concert-hall invites. My once-grand reading schedule was reduced to a lecture in front of four people at a small college in West Virginia and an appearance in a dark corner of a condemned Pittsburgh parking garage during an arts festival. The Greatest Living

American Writer schtick wasn't much of a draw in Appalachia, apparently.

I now found myself waking up most mornings in a drafty townhouse on a transitional block in North Philadelphia. When I wasn't dodging gunfire, the only freelance work I had in front of me was writing the copy for Weight Watchers' new "Men's Program." But I did have an agent. Occasionally, editors still called. The party train might have actually retracked if I hadn't, in the words of Robert Downey Jr. in *Tropic Thunder,* gone "full retard."

Having lost all my connections and privilege, I naturally decided to become the one-man vanguard of a punk rock literary revolution that would take down corporate publishing once and forever. I began spitting water on my audiences and bashing my hardworking peers in the press. Sometimes on stage, I'd tear up books of literary merit, like *Infinite Jest* or *Everything Is Illuminated*, and sometimes I'd set those pages on fire. One night in a Chicago bookstore, I destroyed a copy of *To Kill a Mockingbird* because Mayor Daley had decreed that the whole city should read that book. *Screw Daley and his middlebrow tastes,* I thought. When an interviewer asked me why I was destroying the books, I replied that I just wanted to "fuck shit up." For some reason, Dave Eggers, who was in the process of creating a nationwide network of innovative literary tutoring centers, didn't ask for my help.

I had a happy marriage, a kid on the way, plenty of friends, and a decent adult relationship with my own parents. Yet my bitterness, fear, and horrible attitude persisted. I ripped off my shirt in public and emptied whiskey bottles onto my head. Why was I this angry? How did I become so cynical and self-absorbed, so quickly? After all, I wasn't *born* a total asshole. Once, half a lifetime ago, I'd been in a club called H.U.G.S., recited Dr. King's speeches in public, and loved every human being equally. What had gone wrong? From whence did this Hulk-like behavior spring? I simply didn't know.

The New York Times Book Review covered my second book, a satirical novel about the history of rock-n-roll. The reviewer didn't like it much. He called it "a blown opportunity, a smart premise that its author sabotages with an avalanche of potty humor and a seeming lack of faith in his ability to construct an actual novel." Well that hurt, but not as much as the personal jab the reviewer took, calling me an "ordinary humor dork, yet another doughy, 35-ish white man with a goatee and thinning hair."

That was the worst possible thing anyone could have said about me. Oh, *boo-hoo*, you might think. *Poor wittle baby got a bad review in the* Times. I know. I *know*. In context, though, it hurt a lot. I may not have been The Greatest Living American Writer, but I certainly thought I was better than ordinary. Somehow the world had missed the Pollack point. Whether or not I was a doughy 35ish white man, I could still make my mark. Something unordinary had to lie ahead for me. I couldn't bear the idea of living otherwise.

The night I read that review, I lay in bed next to my wife.

"My hair *is* thinning," I said.

"At least you shaved your goatee," she said.

"He called me ordinary."

I turned over, shoved my face into my pillow, and began pounding the bed with both fists.

"They punished me!" I said. "THEY . . . THEY DE-STROYED ME!!! WHY? WHY? WHY?!"

Never mind that there was no "they" and that no one gave enough of a crap about me to try to plot my destruction. This had gone beyond feeling sorry for myself. Now I despaired for my very life. I'm not being melodramatic when I say that a great chasm had opened at the base of my soul. The confusion, the multiple identities, the very public search for self, it all suddenly exploded, and I felt like I'd been ripped in two, possibly three. All my dreams and hopes had been ruinously perverted. This was low as a human being could possibly get—down, deep, dirty low. I'd become a Robert Johnson song, refracted through the overeducated prism of *This American Life.*

During my usual identity tantrums, Regina sat patiently and waited for the storm to pass. But she could see that this one was more serious than the others; I was actually suffering this time. She rubbed my back soothingly and cooed in my ear. All the grief and anxiety of the past four years poured out of me in a great neurotic wave.

When it was over, I picked my face up out of a viscous puddle of salt water and boogers. I looked up at Regina, sniffling, my eyes lost and pleading.

"What now?" I asked.

"You should do yoga with me," she said.

At the time, Regina and I lived in Austin, Texas, within walking distance of an all-night doughnut shop run by a middle-aged Indian couple. We could sense the doughnuts from our backyard; their odor was sweet enough to overpower the stench of highway diesel, and they tasted even better than they smelled. So we went there a lot. Occasionally, I'd eat a half-dozen maple-glazed before bed, plus a couple of holes, which the owner often gave me as a kind of frequent-stuffer award.

My general state of health had become unhealthy. Because of a less-than-ideal ergonomic work setup, I'd started to walk like Marty Feldman in *Young Frankenstein*, complete with shifting hump. Back pain was my portion and my burden. I'd reached my thirties an exhausted mess of skin tags and moles, little hip tugs, neckaches, and high triglycerides. I could sense whiffs of my stale old-man breath from the future. Middle age, if it hadn't yet quite arrived, had begun to rap on the window of my perception.

Then, in a fortuitous act of real-estate development, a 24-Hour Fitness opened less than a mile away from our house. The choice was clear, in our minds: Join, or die young. We chose the former, and got to like the place pretty well, though late in our membership it strangely transformed into a neon-yellow shrine to Lance Armstrong, with plate-glass reliquary displays that fell just short of manifesting The Great One's testicular X-rays. But the equipment was new and there was a fantastic Kids Club staffed by gorgeous young cheerleaders who never complained when our toddler crapped his pants at the top of the slide.

And they offered yoga classes. Regina had done yoga a few times in the past. She wanted to start again, and she stayed on me about taking classes with her.

"Naaah," I said.

"Come on," Regina said. "It's awesome. Really relaxing."

"Do I have to?"

"It'll be good for your neck and back."

"I don't know."

She swayed her hips back and forth.

"You'll look sex-eeeee . . ." she said. "You'll be a sexy, sexy yoga man."

She said this with so many layers of irony that no one should have been able to take it seriously. But I've always found irony a turn on. So I said, "How much does it cost?"

"It's free with our membership," she said.

Free: the magic word.

"I'll do it," I said.

Our first teacher was a placid-looking woman named Amy, our age or a little younger. She had a kind, pretty face, broad hips, mildly glowing skin, and an easy demeanor. Sitting cross-legged at the front of the room, she put her hands on her knees and spoke calmly and gently. "Close your eyes," she said. "Focus on your breath. Feel it flow in and out of your lungs. Sit up nice and tall. Feel your spine straighten from the base of your tailbone to the crown of your head. Whatever happened before you came into this room doesn't matter, and whatever happens after doesn't matter either. There's only the here and now."

Fair enough, I thought. Lord knows I had plenty of random, useless thoughts and emotions to deposit at the anxiety bank. I didn't mind clearing my mind. But I lacked training, and Amy's words couldn't stop me from twitchily looking around the room like a guy at his first AA meeting. Either I was the only man in Texas who had a free hour at 10 AM on a Wednesday, or guys just didn't do yoga. Everyone else in the room was female. As I sat there in my coffee-stained white T-shirt and my paint-spattered cotton shorts with the "native" Guatemalan pattern embroidered across the hem, I felt self-conscious, hairy, and overly large, an ogre invited to a debutante ball.

The class followed the pattern of most beginning yoga classes: some stretching, some poses, a couple of light back-bends, deep relaxation, and a short meditation. At the time, though, it tasted to me as exotic as a jackfruit milkshake. We pushed back into our first downward dog. It felt like I had bricks in my calves. My flabby hamstrings moaned and my near-arthritic shoulders shuddered. Later, as I creak-ily rose into my first warrior one, my spine crackled like a thick estuarial branch falling off an old tree. My front knee popped unpleasantly.

As the practice continued, my body insulted me in many different ways. I couldn't touch my toes. Bending for-ward over my knees, I caught the faint and unpleasant whiff of my own ass. I hopped and wobbled and stumbled with all the grace of a wounded animal charging through the brush.

Amy wasn't a master, at least not in the gut-straining, semi-didactic way of some of the big-city mega-yogis I've encountered since, but I didn't need a master. I needed someone kind and competent who wouldn't kill me. She explained the simplest poses in very clear language, keep-ing the pace slow and gentle; she was the perfect teacher for beginners. I was kind of enjoying myself; I'd expected poses with flouncy names, like laughing daisy, or bejew-eled vagina, or the infamous happy baby that I'd heard about. Instead, I got masculine ones like warrior and cobra, household objects such as chair and plank, and a variety of ordinary-sounding shapes and animals. Nothing made me blush or shrink into myself with embarrassment. When I finished, I felt worked out but not worn out, sweaty but not disgusting, and much, much calmer. Regina felt the same way. We wanted to do the yoga again.

Our setup at Lance Armstrong 24-Hour Fitness didn't match any form of the yogic ideal. We practiced above the basketball court and next to the spinning center, so we often had to compete with full-volume music scream-ing "DO YOU BELIEVE IN LIFE AFTER LOVE? AFTER LOVE? AFTER LOVE? AFTER LOVE?" This message could, technically, be interpreted as yoga-relevant, but not on repeat for fifty minutes. The space also contained the cleaning-supplies closet, which led to some awkward walk-throughs by the janitorial staff. Because of some obscure gym policy, our teacher wasn't allowed to turn off the lights during *savasana*, which kind of defeated the point since it's hard to transcend your earthly form while baking under a toxically illumined blanket of industrial-strength fluores-cent gym lighting. But Regina and I, lying on our 24-Hour Fitness mats, were at the nascence of our yoga lives, and we didn't really care.

Amy taught twice a week, in the mornings, and there were rarely more than a dozen people in the room. After a few weeks, Regina and I had gained enough confidence to try a supplemental evening class, run by a guy who one friend called "the gay drill sergeant," which wasn't really fair, since the fact that he was gay had no bearing on the in-herent brutality of his class. We'd unwittingly stepped into a den of Power Yoga, and we weren't ready. We found our-selves trapped in a high-octane exercise nightmare, flailing and flopping in a sweaty panic, lost in a senseless flow of arm balances and leg lifts. The gay drill sergeant's class was popular, like forty people popular, so he didn't have time to ride to our aid.

Fifteen minutes into our first session, Regina looked at me, her eyes straining and desperate. She rasped:

"What the fuck is alligator pose?"

Gradually, the practices got a little easier. Not a lot, but enough for us to continue our yogic studies at Lance Armstrong 24-Hour Fitness. The gay drill sergeant suddenly started acting like a yoga teacher instead of an aerobics instructor. He began a weekly series exploring different chakras. At that point I didn't know what a chakra was—very basically, according to traditional Indian medicine, they're spherical energy centers located along different points of the spine—but the progression of the classes became intriguing to me; I began to suspect that there was more to yoga practice than meets the muscular-skeletal system.

One day, he talked about the word *namaste,* usually the last thing said before the end of class. *Namaste,* like *shalom,* is a very useful word that can mean almost anything. He presented it as meaning "my best self honors your best self." Mostly, I was still struggling to make it through my next *vinyasa,* and wasn't spending a lot of time thinking about alternate definitions of Sanskrit vocabulary. But I did already have the concept of my "best self" in my head.

Since I'd started doing yoga, I'd been feeling better physically and even mentally. Still, I was nowhere near my best self. I'd fallen pretty far into the identity pit, and it was going to take me a long time to recover. It occurred to me that my "best self" had actually been most evident during those last two years of high school, when I had a hug for everyone and nothing could stop my train of good feeling. Since then, my life had been a lot more interesting, my world broader, and my experience more complete. But at that moment I could really have used a return to the "best self" of the spring of my adulthood, minus all the late '80s motivational cheese.

As my generation aged, realizing that death was around the corner if not down the block, our habits were turning from self-destructive to self-preserving. All around me, it seemed, people were trying to forestall death, or at least enter the back nine of life with some manner of grace. A friend who had once been a hard-core partier emerged as a holistic acupuncturist. Another reappeared as a shaman in West Virginia. There were amateur herbalists, Pilates teachers-in-training, people who made their own pickles, and organic gardeners. So I started thinking, why not go for that best self again? Yoga seemed like a good candidate for my life raft.

At the same time, the whole concept of finding my best self went against everything for which I stood. It even *sounded* stupid. One of my most hated moments in movie history is when Billy Crystal's wife in *City Slickers* tells his character to "go and find your smile." That sounded like self-absorbed boomer crap to me when I first saw it, and it still does. Yet here I was, at the same basic place in my life as Billy Crystal in *City Slickers*. Instead of trying to find my smile, I was looking for my "best self," but it was still the same damn thing. What if I succeeded? In a couple of years, would I go searching for Curly's Gold?

Nevertheless, I had to put that cynicism aside, at least

partially, because I found myself wanting to go deeper into the yoga. Like a freshly made vampire, I'd only just begun to test the limits of my thirst. Yoga was about to become the organizing principle of my existence. Also, much to the chagrin of non-yogis I knew, it became pretty much the only thing about which I ever wanted to talk. In the walk of life, I'd stepped in a big pile of yoga doo, and nothing could get it off my sole. Or my soul.

2

Smoothly, and with Ease

A few months later, because I wanted to raise my son in a clean, unpretentious place full of genuine people who exuded human kindness, I moved my family to Los Angeles. Following a long tradition of American hack writers with limited financial prospects, I sought to court the affections of the Hollywood establishment. My high-concept parenting memoir *Alternadad* was nearing publication, and I sensed an impending windfall of glamour and riches. Soon, my fascinating life story would be made into a hilarious, popular movie starring Ben Stiller. No one close to me would ever want for anything ever again. It was all about to turn around.

We rented a house off Craig's List. The people who'd checked it out in proxy wrote us: "If you don't take this house, we will." Despite this positive review, the fact that we couldn't afford to fly to L.A. to house shop should have been a sign that we weren't exactly about to settle in Laurel Canyon.

As we turned off the highway and entered our new neighborhood, Regina and I looked around us and realized it was just like our old neighborhood, only more crowded, twice as expensive, and about eight times as ominous. In Austin, though we'd lived down the block from a day-labor center, the same block where someone was stabbed through the heart with a coat hanger in broad daylight, at least our neighbors were warm, friendly, and fun. We were part of a community, and felt loved and protected, and we didn't yet live on a street, as we would in L.A., that had long been the site of entrenched gang warfare. Most days, there were few signs of that, though occasionally a windowless white van would squeal by at 60 MPH, followed by two angry police cars. The house to our west was owned by elderly sisters who refused to speak with us after they learned we hadn't voted for George W. Bush; in the house to our east lived a large Mexican family that refused to speak with us, period. Every time our gazes met as we got into our cars in our respective driveways, the patriarch looked at me as though I were a gentrifier from Planet Douchebag. Regina and I moaned regretfully to each other. If crappy housing choices were horses, we'd have owned a stable of champions. But they weren't, and instead we rented a crappy house.

We were alone.

One January night, my family sat on the couch, shutters drawn to the world, gloomily watching television. A terrible, freezing rainstorm had driven us inside. We cuddled for warmth and friendship. There was a knock at the door.

Regina and I looked at each other, a little annoyed and a little fearful. The week we moved to L.A., Regina had answered the door to reveal a one-armed woman who was asking for money to benefit the family of a teenaged girl who'd been slain in some random act of gang violence. Regina gave her a dollar. I placed a panicked call to the neighborhood beat officer. This was a scam, he assured us. All the gang violence had moved either six blocks to the east or to the south. Our block was full of "stakeholders." It was where the gang members' mothers lived, and the gang members didn't mess with their mothers.

So we'd learned to be skeptical of knocks. But on nights like this, even scam artists stayed home. I got up.

Through the slats of our door-length plastic blinds, I saw the Frenchwoman who lived in the house behind us. A PhD candidate in bioengineering at USC, she made a good neighbor: quiet, rarely home, and prone to taking weeklong surfing trips to Hawaii. We were friendly enough with her, though she never did thank us for the holiday cookies we'd left on her doorstep.

"I have a leetle problem," she said.

"What?" I said.

"Eet's a dog."

She opened the door further. Behind her was a medium-size dog that had once been some kind of terrier. Its white fur had been torn in chunks from its torso, revealing a hideous vista of red-raw skin and sores and eminently visible bones. The rest of the dog was filthy and soaking wet. It looked ready to die.

"Eet followed me home," she said. "I don't know much about dogs."

"We have a dog!" I said proudly.

"I know," she said. "That's why I'm asking for your help."

Our dog was a neckless Boston Terrier named Hercules. His hobbies included eating cat barf, licking my ankles under the bedcovers, and moping on the couch. When we took him for walks, we had to lift him over puddles because he was afraid of the water. Compared with the other dogs in this neighborhood, hungry-looking Pit Bulls and Boxers who spent their entire lives shitting in concrete lots enclosed by rusting wrought iron bars, Hercules was really more Muppet than dog. Owning him hardly qualified me as an expert in canine care.

Still, I'd been feeling useless, neutered, and alone since we'd moved to town. This seemed like the perfect mission to break my slump. A great surge of heroism and duty welled in my chest. I began barking orders.

"Regina! Get me some dog food! And a bowl! No! *Two* bowls! And a towel! And some treats and some doggie shampoo! We're gonna clean up this mutt!"

The French girl left with the dog. A few minutes later, I walked through the rain to the house at the back of the property, where she lived. It already smelled like dog throughout.

"Eet's a he," she said. "I looked."

The stray cowered in her kitchen. When I offered him doggie treats, he just looked confused, like he'd been hungry so long that he'd forgotten the purpose of food. So I skipped that step, picked him up in a towel, and carried him to the bathroom. Then I placed him in the tub, soaked him with water from a cup, and scrubbed him down with Johnson's Baby Shampoo. He behaved himself. At least the water was warm. When we were done, he still smelled like death, but at least it was clean death.

"Now what do I do?" asked my neighbor.

"Call a vet?" I said.

For some reason, instead of making the call herself, she handed me the phone book. I dialed the Eagle Rock Emergency Animal Hospital.

"Yes, hello," I said. "I have a dog here. I found . . . well, actually, my neighbor found him on the street and took him home and then I gave him a bath. Where should I send him?"

"You need to get in touch with the Humane Society," said the man on the other line.

"OK."

"And, because you handled the dog, you might have mange."

"What?"

"Mange," he said, flatly. "Scabies. You should check with your doctor in two weeks. It usually doesn't set in for a month to six weeks. And if you have it, then everyone you come into contact with will get it, too."

"Are you saying I shouldn't touch anybody for a month?"

"Just to be safe."

"Mange?" I said. "Are you *sure* I have mange?"

"Go to your doctor," he said. "You have mange."

This seemed impossible. I'd bathed the dog with disinfectant shampoo and had washed my hands afterward. I've come into contact with stray dogs many times. And yet mange is not on the list of diseases I've contracted. I hung up the phone, said a hurried, "I've got to go," to my neighbor, and ran home in a panic.

"We have mange," I said to Regina.

"What?"

"You need to take off all your clothes and put them in the washer."

"You're kidding."

"Do it! NOW! And take off Elijah's clothes, too! And Hercules's collar!"

"Oh, come on."

"Dammit, Regina," I said. "We have mange! Mange!"

"Nooooo!" said my son. "I'm cold. I don't want to take off my clothes!"

Though we quickly determined that Hercules's heartworm medication protects him from mange, and we also learned that while people *can* contract mange, it's an entirely different disease than the one that afflicts dogs, that evening still found the three of us in our underwear, huddled together, shivering, afraid of having contracted mange, and watching *Monsters, Inc.* A year ago at this time I'd had lots of friends, a house that I owned, and a relaxed lifestyle that caused me a relatively small amount of stress. Now I found myself surrounded by enemies in a small rental house in a city that has destroyed thousands of men far greater than me. What the hell were we doing in Los Angeles?

This was a job for yoga.

I'd read an article in the *LA Weekly* where a long-time
teacher said, "Los Angeles today is to yoga what Paris in the
1920s was to literature and art . . . Some of the best teachers
in the world are centered here, and this is a highly creative
moment." Of course, that same article described how the
best elements of L.A. yoga were being destroyed by suspect
corporate business practices and the rampant egos of high-
powered mega-yogis. But what did I care? It was Paris in
the 20s, and I was actually there! I needed to find a studio
where I could continue my transcendental education, the
search for my best self.

I subscribed to a free email newsletter called *Chill Out
LA*, which turned out to be mostly listings for wellness spas
in Santa Monica and therefore almost totally useless to me,
since I intended to visit the West Side of town about as often
as I visited West Virginia. But about a month after arriving,
I got an email about Karuna Yoga on Hillhurst Avenue, in
the heart of the Marginally Employed Hipster with Yuppie
Aspirations District. It was offering a great ten-class deal
for new students.

A quick browse revealed no "This place is horrible,
rude, and dirty" entries on Yelp or Citysearch, though there
was a warning that "they will expire your classes on you."
This didn't bother me; the thought of paying for something
that I don't use fills me with pure existential dread. I don't
even allow myself to have overdue library books, so there's
no way I'd get saddled with expired yoga classes. I called
upon the good folks at Karuna Yoga.

The studio was small and quiet and pleasant, candlelit
with a nice mild incense smell and soothing, dark yellow

walls and a sheer gold curtain at the front of the room. After class, in an outdoor seating area, they offered mint tea and organic animal cookies. A sign faced the street, but the studio could only be reached by walking into an alley past an overpriced ladies-who-lunch joint called The Alcove. Karuna trended small, subtle, and neighborhoody, just how I liked my businesses. I ponied up for the ten classes and prepared to see the light. The search for my best self, for now, would continue here.

When I went to the studio for my first class, there was only one other student. The teacher spent all night comparing me to her, unfavorably. The more she criticized me, the more nervous I got. I stumbled around in despair.

"Sometimes it's better not to try something until you know what you're doing," said the teacher.

Later, she added, "Maybe you should sit down until we get to a pose you can actually do."

Those are the types of careless, errant comments that make people quit yoga forever, and I was feeling a tad vulnerable.

After class, I walked down the street, softly moaning to myself. My life was a lie, my bank account dwindling, my online enemies legion, my career a fraud. Now even yoga had betrayed me. The gods mocked me cruelly!

The other student walked past and saw me daubing my eyes.

"Oh, dear," she said. "Sorry about that."

"I'm doing the best I can!" I whined.

"I know," she said kindly, as though she'd taken classes with out of shape, insecure Jewish men before. "You should try Patty."

My first class with Patty marked the true dawn of my yoga dorkdom. The studio advertised her class as "*hatha* yoga," but that's just the generic term for any physical form of yoga. Walking into a *hatha* yoga class in L.A. is like signing up for an acting lesson. You have about equal odds of either learning something vital from a highly qualified professional or getting sucked into a strange "technique" crafted by an egomaniacal lunatic. Fortunately for me, Patty fit the former category. She combined the heat-generating rigor of *vinyasa* with the intense pose holding of *iyengar* with little dashes of *ashtanga* thrown in to torture us. At the time, I had no idea what any of that meant, but she mixed it up a lot, and I always learned how to do something new.

Patty gave off a mellow, mature, serene vibe, possibly because she was from New Mexico. Everyone I've ever known from there has been pretty chill. Regardless, she was a great teacher who never made me feel bad. There was no right or wrong in yoga class, she said. There was only the practice. *Yeah,* I thought. *The practice. I get it now.* On one memorable morning, she gave us the only purely physical instruction from the *Yoga Sutras:* "Find a comfortable seat." That's always been a special skill of mine. If her second instruction had been "Eat three dozen extra-hot chicken wings while watching the opening night of NBA League Pass," I would have followed her to the ends of the universe. But those were long odds.

To my relief, Patty never chanted, but sometimes at the end of class she would read this little piece of Buddhist *metta* meditation:

"May you feel protected and safe/May you feel contented

and pleased/May your body support you with strength/May your life unfold smoothly, and with ease."

Since I currently felt or experienced none of those things, I found the philosophy appealing.

Like most teachers at Karuna, Patty kept the loud, hip music to a minimum, though she did charm Regina and I when she played the theme from *A Charlie Brown Christmas* during holiday time. Her mixes sometimes included Crowded House songs. This was because her husband sometimes plays guitar with Crowded House. I now lived in a social environment where "my nanny is Scarlett Johansson's best friend" is considered an acceptable social gambit. Therefore, I tried several times to deploy "my yoga teacher's husband is in Crowded House," to little effect. "My accountant used to be the drummer for The Circle Jerks," also true, never got me invited to parties either.

Patty's classes quickly became the highlight of my week, a centering force in a town where everyone else is out to destroy you whether they know you or not. She attracted a generally noncompetitive mix of struggling actresses, marginally employed screenwriters, struggling actresses trying to become marginally employed screenwriters, someone who worked for the Beverly Hills Chamber of Commerce, a very nice psychiatrist, and the occasional tall dude with gnarly tattoos. Regina often came with me, and sometimes she didn't.

One Reginaless morning, Patty had us do handstands against the wall, with the help of our partners. I was so eager to invert that I didn't see who'd been assigned to me. My hands pressed against the wall and I drew my legs up until they were in a *V* shape. I looked through my legs and saw another pair of legs, presumably male, standing upright.

"I've got you," a voice said.

I kicked my legs. A hand grabbed either ankle and helped me into my inversion. When I looked up, I was staring upside-down at the smiling face of Gedde Watanabe, the guy who'd played Long Duk Dong in *Sixteen Candles*. I really, really wanted to say "Oh sexy giiiiiiirlfriend," but in L.A., you had to be cool around celebrity, no matter how minor. So instead, I said, "What's happening, hot stuff?"

No, I didn't say that, either, however much I wanted to. Instead, I just said "thanks, man," and when it came time to give Long Duk Dong a leg lift, I returned the favor.

One morning, I found myself on the mat next to an attractive Czech model, which ordinarily would have been a cause for celebration. But she was one bossy Slav. She'd been at this yoga gig longer than I had, and she saw things in my posture she didn't like.

I got a little correction. Then I got another. By the time she'd corrected me five times, I was sighing. At the sixth correction, I picked up my mat and left the room, huffing audibly. I sat outside and murmured: "I can't fucking believe it . . . who the fuck does she think she is, telling *me* how to handle *my* yoga practice? I know what I'm doing!" It was the kind of thing that I'd be grumbling to myself in twenty years as I pushed a shopping cart containing all my possessions down the less-touristy end of Hollywood Boulevard.

After class, Patty asked Regina if I felt OK.

"Yeah," Regina said. "He just does things like that sometimes."

That evening, I wrote Patty an email, saying I didn't want anyone but the teacher talking to me in class. She understood where I was coming from, but defended the student's "youthful exuberance, well-meaning intentions and cultural differences." That sounded a lot more appetizing than my aging cynicism, complete lack of interest in others, and lifetime of enthusiastic immersion in a culture that encourages you to look out for number one. Clearly, my best self was miles down the road.

But my physical yoga, at least, had improved, or so I thought. Near the end of practice a couple of weeks later, Patty told us to prepare for *urdhva dhanurasana*, or, for those of you who don't know Sanskrit, upward-facing bow pose. Around certain yoga parts, the pose is more commonly called wheel, but whatever the name, it's a classic—a real fucking doozy. Going wheel was a major yoga signpost for me. Fully expressed, it looks super freaky, the kind of backbend that, when you don't do yoga, you look at and say, "Man, those yoga people are crazy."

I'd gotten to the point where I could push up pretty much every time, and I was feeling confident. So my palms planted, and I rose. Patty told us to try moving our heels closer to our butts. On the way there, one of my heels skidded. Then one of my arms flipped out to the side. I crashed to the mat and heard a popping sound in my left shoulder. This wasn't a pleasant pop, like the sound your hips make when tilting into triangle pose. It didn't feel like the sweet release I get when I twist around and crack my lower vertebrae. Instead, I felt hot, fresh pain in a place where I'd never felt pain before. My face must have contorted as though I'd been stabbed, because Patty said,

"Don't do anything else. Just get some ice on that shoulder immediately."

The studio didn't have ice, so I moped next door to The Alcove, got a little cold baggie, and then went back to the benches to wait for Regina to finish her practice. The shoulder hurt. My arm hung limply at my side; I could only lift it up about halfway before the burn hit. I'd been totally gimped.

In some ways, it was a victory that I'd actually gotten to a point where I could inflict that kind of pain on myself. For much of my life, my body had felt like it belonged to someone else. As a kid, I often wrote stories or drew comics imagining myself as a floating brain in a jar, disconnected from the concerns of corporeal reality. Probably, I watched too much *Doctor Who*, but the fact remained that I felt ill at home in my skin. I didn't learn to ride a bike until I was six-teen, and I had trouble telling my right hand from my left. More often than not, I dropped things. The only sport I'd ever been any good at was racquetball, largely practiced by spastic rich old men wearing goggles. Yoga, in addition to being the one true path to my best self, was the first physical activity in which I'd made progress since around puberty, and it was about time that I found something to replace, or at least supplement, my daily masturbation practice. When I did yoga, I found myself moving with a modicum of grace, strength, and calm. My brain no longer floated in an imaginary jar. Therefore, I had to recover and return to my practice immediately.

But how could I, with my bad shoulder? What if I needed Tommy John surgery? It sometimes took baseball pitchers *years* to move past that, and they get paid millions of dollars to sit in whirlpools while continually being massaged by hirsute professional trainers. Whirlpools were beyond my budget; I couldn't even get my bathtub to drain properly. As the days passed and my shoulder continued to ache, that old familiar depression began to cloud my brain.

I went to a progressive sports medicine clinic in Westwood, where I saw doctors and chiropractors and various other special interest body manipulators. They poked and pulled and twisted. Somehow, by ordering up an analysis of the vitamin content of my blood, they even got me out of paying my deductible. These were some doctors! They determined that I had a rotator cuff muscle strain, related to an imbalance between my right and left sides. I'd been favoring my right knee for years, ever since a drunken college student had smashed it with a whiskey bottle in a hot tub. It was time to put that night behind me.

Over a few visits, the staff massaged me, rubbed me with cream, and stimulated the damaged cuff with electricity. They gave me an exercise regimen. I took home a length of dark-green rubber tubing tied into loops at both ends. I put one loop around my wrist, and one around my foot, and did various exercises where I pumped my arm into different positions. These hurt pretty bad at first. Gradually they hurt less, but I wanted them to hurt until they hurt in the good way. I wanted the pain. I wanted the work. I was going to get my ass on that mat again.

I had the eye of the motherfucking tiger.

A month later, I returned to the studio. Nobody had noticed I'd been gone, but that didn't matter. I knew the moderately bumpy side road I'd taken to get back.

Midway through class, we got ready to do a tough arm

balance. Patty looked at me, concerned. I waved her off, and she gave me a nonchalant nod. I was back, baby, all the way. I thought: *Let the cymbals clang and the gongs strike in celebration. My story will serve as inspiration to fallen yogis everywhere. Send out an OM to the world: Nothing can stop my spiritual progress now.*

Maybe I'd even start taking more than one class a week.

Another popular teacher at Karuna was Tanya. She mostly taught in the *anusara* style. This form of yoga started in 1996, making it newer than some of my pets. It revolves around heart-opening poses, and it's quickly spread around the country like some sort of good-feeling yoga virus. If your teacher's under, say, forty years old, you have high odds of getting saddled with at least a little *anusara* philosophy.

Tanya's classes started at 7:45 PM, so getting there was a challenge. I couldn't often say, "Have fun putting the kid to bed, dear. I'm off to yoga!" if I still wanted my testicles attached to my body the next morning. But after my difficult rehab, my wife took mercy.

One night, finally, I went to Tanya's class. She had a degree in yoga therapy from the excellent program at Loyola Marymount. Her alignments were precise and invigorating. I could feel my warrior two improving markedly under her watch. We held our poses for a long time, and it hurt; if your teacher makes your quadriceps quiver, you're in good hands. Oh, how my yoga was evolving! My body and my mind were changing, becoming something grander and higher!

During the cool down, Tanya told us to draw our knees by our ears. We grabbed our feet with our hands and rocked gently from side to side. This was happy baby pose. My body felt free and loose, totally relaxed in every way.

A murmur emanated from my guts, and an airy whoosh moved through my intestines.

I then uncorked the sloppiest, wettest fart of my life, a desperate five-second bleat of sweet relief. The sound seemed to bounce around the walls of the studio like a rubber ball thrown at maximum velocity. I followed this with a series of three little toots, duckling farts chasing after their mother. It was like the campfire scene in *Blazing Saddles* except that, instead of cowboys, hot chicks in Spandex surrounded me, and I was the only one farting.

"*Oh, yeah,*" Tanya said. "That's it."

My fart had been so strong that even my *teacher* felt relief. I quaked with humiliation and self-hatred.

"Oh my God," I said. "I'm such a Jew."

The class roared in appreciative laughter, which made me even more nervous. Really, what did Judaism have to do with farting? *My* comment could be explained away by self-loathing, but what was *their* excuse? Were all yogis secret anti-Semites?

Regardless, from then on, whenever I went to Tanya's class I couldn't contain my flatulence. I ripped and hissed and tooted. There were silent deadlies and noisy, odorless farts. I farted while standing, sitting, and lying down. The sorrowful people next to me tried to stare stoically ahead and focus on their practice, but I knew they were thinking: Who is this hairy, ass-blowing Heeb next to me, and how can I prevent him from ever coming to class again?

It got bad enough that I began to develop a theory of yoga farting, and even a strategy. Though the noisy farts smelled the least, they also provided the most distraction to the other students. If I felt a loud one moving toward my anus, I tightened my perineal muscles and willed it away. This is known, in yoga, as the *mulabahnda*, or pelvic lock. Did the first yogis introduce it as a fart retainer? I suppose people *did* fart three thousand years ago. *Possibly,* I thought, *my theory of yoga farting had ancient roots.*

If I absolutely had to cut loose, I tried to let it out slowly and subtly, with a nice hiss. That didn't always work, though, and little plopping sounds would emerge. These worked best in moments of transition, from sitting to standing or vice-versa, or when our teacher had us move our mats to the wall. If at all possible, I liked for my farts to get lost in a wave of sound. Therefore, the best time to fart, if I absolutely had to, was during the part of the class where we said "OM." As a beautiful chorus of human voices (including mine) harmonized as one, my colon expanded and contracted, discharging useless gases. I sent them out to the cosmos as an extra blessing, a karmic bonus.

Then I realized the farts were mostly preventable.

One night before Tanya's class, I sat down for dinner with my family. As I ate, I looked at my plate. I'd devoured half a chicken, a huge helping of mashed potatoes with buttermilk, and a hefty serving of broccoli. No wonder I was farting during yoga class. That night, I had to deploy my usual strategies, but before Tanya's class the following week, I just ate a couple of carrots to settle my stomach.

I did the entire practice without even the mildest gastrointestinal disturbance. My body felt free and loose. It twisted and rose and fell with great ease. Free of worrying about my farts, my mind could think about higher things, like what I was going to eat for dinner after class.

At some point, Tanya had us hook up with a partner for an assisted handstand. I got assigned to some dude I'd never met before. My spirit flowed freely and exuberantly. Also, my left leg flung out and smacked him in the face. To his credit, he let me down gently before he grabbed his face and yelled "OW!"

"Oh my God," I said. "I'm so sorry!"

"It's OK," he said.

The teacher came over.

"What happened?" she asked. "Did you get kicked?"

"Yeah," he said.

I could see that he was going to get a fat lip out of the deal.

Tanya said, "I've been kicked before. It's no fun."

That ended the situation. I didn't say goodbye to the guy after class. No one mentioned the kick. It was like it had never happened. Though it stayed in *my* mind, I realized later that, except for probably the guy I'd kicked, no one else on earth remembered the incident. This wasn't like martial arts, where you're *supposed* to kick guys in the face. Sure, you shouldn't make a habit of kicking your fellow yogis in the face, but if you do, it doesn't matter. In yoga, I could kick a guy in the face, and no one cared. Wicked.

3

The Crystalline Center of the Hard Core

A year passed, and then a few more months. I got into the Writer's Guild of America, which meant decent health insurance for the first time in nearly a decade. Soon, a TV development deal followed. My workdays now involved hammering out story beats with co-writers at a house in Sherman Oaks. We traded in our station wagon, and then I was another Prius-driving asshole.

Our housing situation also changed. Elijah's kindergarten year approached. Thanks again to Craigslist, we found a rental house in a nicer neighborhood with better schools, within walking distance of grocery stores, restaurants, bars, a public library, Robek's Smoothies, and Karuna Yoga. The skies had brightened over Pollackville. I started running out of reasons to feel sorry for myself. We were movin' on up, to the not-as-far East Side.

Ah, but in Los Angeles, every silver lining contains a cloud. The Writer's Guild of America voted to stage an industry-crippling strike. Overnight, my workdays became walking around Paramount Studios with a picket sign from 10 AM to 2 PM, sucking down truck fumes and having conversations with retired *Star Trek* writers, and then going home, burying my head in my hands at the kitchen table, and wondering how I was going to pay rent on the new house, which was 40 percent more expensive than the old one.

Also, the house itself, despite its location, location, location, was proving to have some major cracks in the façade. My workspace was a dusty, windowless basement connected to the garage, which seemed romantic at first, but proved less than pleasant when it filled with toxic leaf blower fumes and when our landlord, a friendly but epically cheap retired high school teacher, advised me to put all my possessions up on bricks because it would probably flood down there when it rained. This didn't prove to be a problem when we found ourselves suffering through a record heat wave, drought, and terrifying fire season. Sunlight blazed through our thoroughly sealed floor-to-ceiling living room window, driving the interior temperature near triple digits. We didn't have air conditioning. When we opened the windows, it didn't take long before all our possessions were coated with a fine layer of soot, ash, and grime.

Our two-block proximity to a major urban high school also proved a problem, as the former tenant had stopped by to warn us. Two months before she'd moved out, a kid had been shot on her lawn. Then I, too, got shot. One night while walking the dog in the hills, a carful of Armenian teenagers buzzed by and nailed me in the shoulder with a BB. Fortunately, I was wearing a leather jacket and barely felt it, but the three-year-old down the street, who got pegged in the throat, and the old lady up the hill, who took it in the belly, weren't so fortunate.

Our new next door neighbor was another constant bother: a batty hag who, when she wasn't hanging out her laundry while wearing hideous thigh-length muumuus, was screaming orders at her part-time house servant, a beleaguered-looking fourteen-year-old Mexican boy. Her attempts to act neighborly fell flat, such as the time she barged through our front door with a copy of *The Bridge to Terabithia,* saying that she thought Elijah would enjoy watching it as long as we got it back to the Video Hut on Hyperion by 7 PM so she didn't have to pay a late fee. Another time, she came aknockin' to ask if I could drive her to Universal Studios. Even though she offered me $10, I declined.

The strike ended. My deal collapsed. We pondered breaking our lease and making a run for my parents' house in Phoenix. I needed yoga more than ever.

Patty sent out an email to her students saying that she was going to start teaching a class every other Sunday at a "lovely Los Feliz home." After the class, there'd be brunch. This sounded nice to me. I'd been looking for somewhere to practice on Sundays, and I'm always a sucker for a food bribe. I pictured a lovely *asana* practice on a sunlit porch followed by unlimited bagels, lox, biscuits, gravy, and shrimp. Now I know that the words "yoga" and "brunch" together only guarantee you fruit. You have to pray for protein.

That Sunday morning, I announced:

"I'm off to yoga practice."

"You are not," Regina said.

"Yes I am," I said. "And you can't stop me."

"I wouldn't dream of it," she said.

"Yoga?" said my son. "Again?"

"Afterward, you can have ice cream," I said.

"OK," he said.

"What do *I* get?" asked Regina.

"You can also have ice cream."

"OK," she said.

This being Los Angeles, I *drove* three blocks to the lovely home. I'd imagined something with at least three bedrooms, floor-to-ceiling bookshelves, and a radio permanently tuned to *Car Talk,* but it turned out to be a one-bedroom apartment in a small complex on Rowena. The door to the apartment was unlocked. I opened it, and my yoga practice changed forever.

Patty wasn't teaching that day. Instead, Mara was in charge, a bit younger than me, lithely compact, dark haired, with olive skin so healthy looking, it almost shined. She lived in the apartment with a longhaired orange cat named Sampson. Her studio, hOM Yoga, comprised the front room. It was meticulously clean and dark; it contained no furniture except a few pillows and a corner shelf of books about yoga and Buddhism. She'd painted aphorisms in beautiful cursive lettering all around the room, on the top of the wall just below the ceiling. One that consistently caught my attention over the subsequent weeks read, "you are not leaving, you are arriving, you are not leaving, you are arriving." Three other students sat on their mats, waiting for class. They were all women.

"Hey," I said. "I'm one of Patty's students."

"Patty only teaches every other Sunday," Mara said, adjusting her nifty red-framed hipster glasses.

"Oh," I said. "I heard there was brunch."

"Only the first week of every month."

"Oh."

"But it's really great that you came," she said. "Isn't it, ladies?"

The ladies all agreed that it was great.

We had a lovely practice, without brunch. Afterward, I talked to Mara a little bit. A former stage actress, she'd decided to pursue an even *less* profitable career as a yoga teacher. She'd started hOM in 2005, after having been studio manager at Karuna for several years and leaving in some obscure dispute that I didn't want to know very much about. Mara referred to hOM as "underground yoga," operating quietly and serenely outside of what she considered a toxic nexus of West Side yoga rock stars and fashion trends. She was a one-stop shop of Eastern culture goodness, offering daily yoga classes, Thai yoga massage, tarot readings, and weekly takeaway vegan and vegetarian cooking. She also performed *kirtan,* Indian devotional singing, in a group called Anaam, and she sometimes used the walls of her apartment as an art gallery. She was way more earnest than most of the people I knew, but I felt relatively at ease around her, even trusting. *This,* I thought, *was a real yoga person.*

She said, "We're starting a morning Ashtanga practice here tomorrow. You should come by."

I got invited to so few things that I would have been interested even if she'd said "a bunch of us are getting together tomorrow to nail ourselves to crosses. Wanna come?"

"Sure!" I said.

When I got home, Regina asked, "How was class?"

"I'm starting an Ashtanga practice tomorrow," I said.

Though my wife had brought me to yoga in the first place, and though she'd placed her mat alongside me during my first months in L.A., she'd gradually been drifting away from the practice. "I'm finding my spiritual center in other ways," she said when I harangued her. These included studying crop circles, reading books on paganism and shamanism, meditating with crystals, emailing with alien-abduction expert Whitley Strieber, and doing free online consultations with a woman who helped people determine the identity of their animal spirit guides. Regina's was a snow leopard. In less than two years, we'd transformed into a couple of bona-fide California fruitcakes.

"Whatever," she said. "I'm getting pretty sick of yoga."

"Not me!" I said.

"How much is that going to cost, anyway?"

"A hundred bucks a month."

"A hundred bucks!!!!"

But considering that drop-in yoga classes easily run $20 now, this seemed to me like more than a bargain. It was almost yoga robbery. Besides, I'd been eyeing Ashtanga for a while. A trusted friend of mine, who'd been a yogini longer than I'd even known yoga existed, swore that Ashtanga was the only true yoga. It eschewed all the airy-fairy bullshit, and it was tougher to master than anything else.

"I don't know," I said. "I've taken some pretty hard yoga classes."

"Yeah," my friend said, "but in Ashtanga they sit on your back until you scream in pain."

"Well," I said. "That *does* sound appealing."

There are four major paths of yoga, as described in ancient texts. Any one of them, practiced correctly, can get you to that elusive total union of body, mind, and spirit. The first, *karma* yoga, is for the person of action. The action-type persons who practice it, say the philosophers, must behave selflessly, without any thought of reward or return. The second type, *bhakti* yoga, is for persons of emotion, religious types who like to pray and spread good feelings of joy and compassion. *Gnana* (or *Jnana*) yoga is all about self-inquiry and self-knowledge. It's very intense, and the hardest kind of yoga to practice. "The Gnana-yogi uses his own mind-body as a laboratory," says Gudjon Bergmann, a yoga teacher whose website I'm cribbing from as I write this. "His main goal is to see beyond that which is not real. The yogi concept of unreal is closely related to the concept of permanence. That which is real is permanent, that which is unreal is impermanent." I think we all can relate.

If I had to pick, I'd say that my yoga, at that point, was about 80 percent *karma*, 20 percent *gnana*. The Ashtanga yoga system that I was about to practice, however, kicked that right in the butt. Ashtanga is also known as *raja* yoga, the yoga of kings, the highest form of practice. In Sanskrit, Ashtanga translates as "eight limbs," which is why you see so many tree metaphors on the walls of yoga studios. The limbs are: ethical observances, positive disciplines, posture, *pranayama* (which translates as "life force control," but for our purposes we'll just call it "breathing"), sense control, concentration, meditation, and enlightenment. They don't have to be practiced in order, thank God. Most Westerners find their way into yoga through the third limb, *asana,* or posture. This is what we know as *hatha,* or physical yoga. When practiced in Ashtanga, it's tough as shit.

In her 2000 *New Yorker* article on the topic, Rebecca Mead called Ashtanga "a system of practice and belief which embraces meditation and breath-control techniques, and includes directives for ethical behavior. But the distinguishing characteristic of Ashtanga is a set of extremely demanding physical postures, or *asanas,* that are performed in a linked, fluid series and are accompanied by a focused pattern of breathing." Ashtanga is "hard-core yoga," she wrote, and dedicated Ashtangis are the "crystalline center of the hard core." It's a progressive practice, meaning you start out doing basically nothing, and then the teacher gives you a few more poses, or sometimes also takes poses away, and then you keep going for the rest of your life because there are six series and all kinds of crazy variations and eventually you learn how to walk backwards on your hands with your head between your legs.

One of the major problems with Ashtanga, I quickly learned, is that it's preferably done early in the morning, a time of day that should be reserved for pulling a pillow over your head while your child shrieks in your ear for you to call up an episode of Spongebob on the TiVo. Ideally, you should finish your practice by 6 AM, but even Mara couldn't get up that early. Instead, she opened her home on Mondays and Wednesdays from 7 to 10 AM for self-guided practice. People could come and go any time within that frame, which meant I was usually only practicing alongside two or three others. She called the class "Morning Mysore," Mysore being the city in India where the family of the late Sri K. Patthabi Jois operates the official Ashtanga Institute. As I progressed, I came to realize why the word "sore" was in the city's name.

After a couple of sessions where I could barely stand upright for fifteen minutes before collapsing, my practice stabilized. It went like this: bend over, rise up, jump back, push up, swoop forward, downward dog, rinse, repeat, more forward bending, grabbing your big toe with thumb and forefinger, bend over, rise up, jump back, arms up, arms parallel, tilt forward, back up, and so on, through many permutations. I held all of these poses for five deep breaths, where I closed my mouth, constricted my throat, and emitted a deep, raspy hiss through my nose. This was *Ujjayi*, the official breath of the Ashtanga system, which must be meticulously coordinated with your practice because when you control your breath, you control your body. It makes you sound like Darth Vader going through puberty.

Next came four intense forward bends, my legs spread far apart, my hands alternately on the floor, at my hips, clasped behind my back, and grabbing my big toes. Balancing followed, where I hooked my big toe and extended my right leg forward, then to the side, then held it straight up while letting go of the toe. After I finished this, I did some time in tree and chair and both warriors.

And that ended my warm up. From there, I proceeded to the "primary series," various seated contortions, bends, and lifts of increasingly impossible degrees. When I started, I did about two poses before I got sent to the "finishing sequence" of backbends, shoulder stands, and a few cross-legged, seated poses before the sweet mercies of *savasana*. After about a month of practice, I'd added a couple more poses, but it wasn't exactly going fast. There were always corrections to be made.

On Fridays at 8 AM, Mara led the entire class in doing the Ashtanga primary series together. This usually ended with me feeling like I'd gotten crushed in an elephant stampede. After class, I spent the rest of my day with my head turned to the ceiling while I tried to remember to wipe the drool off my chin. Enlightenment, indeed. Imagine going to the dentist every day to get the same tooth filled until he gets the filling right, except he never gets it right, and you have to keep going back. Ashtanga was like being in the yoga army. But like the Army, it made a man of me, without the part when you get beaten in the shower with a pillowcase full of soap if you make a mistake. Just as there's no "I" in "team," there's no "team" in Ashtanga.

I persisted through the summer. Like lifting weights at the gym, Ashtanga could be really tedious, but there was no arguing with the results. When I took non-Ashtanga classes at other studios, the postures suddenly seemed a lot easier and calmer, and I was able to push myself deeper. On off days, I started doing the sequence by myself at home. Muscles began to appear where they'd never appeared before. It increasingly seemed like I would reach age forty without looking like the Comic Book Guy from *The Simpsons*. For the first time in a long time, maybe ever, I actually looked like a man, or what I thought a man *should* look like.

Once it became public knowledge that yoga had taken over my life, people started asking if I'd learned any new sexual positions, largely because they wanted to make fun of me. Someone asked if I was now more "bendy." Another said, "so, are you like having that Tantric sex stuff for twelve straight hours at a time, you know, like Sting and Trudy?"

Well, I'd definitely grown more agile and more flexible. I wasn't flopping around like a decked marlin in bed, and didn't find myself wheezing for breath when I was done. But it's not like Regina and I continually writhed in sweet *Kama Sutra* sexual congress, tenderly moving our outstretched hands in a circle while facing each other in half-moon pose. Allow me to quote Sting from a revealing interview he did with a British tabloid: "Yes, you can have sex for six hours, but it includes dinner, a movie and maybe a lot of begging! Tantra is a well-documented science, it's not just about sex. It's a devotional exercise to express adoration. Sex is a sacred act and incredible fun."

For the first time since the release of *Synchronicity*, I found myself agreeing with Sting. Let me add that I actually hadn't studied Tantra, at all, so I definitely wasn't having rock-star intercourse. Plus, if Sting, a physically impeccable world-famous billionaire musician who owns most of Scotland, has to beg his wife for sex, where did that leave guys like me? By the time Regina and I got done with dinner and a movie, all we cared about was rushing home so we didn't have to pay the babysitter an extra ten bucks, which didn't really put us in the mood to make sexy time.

Certain things did change. When you spend ten hours a week or more doing intense yoga, you continually contract and flex your perineum muscles, and the area between your testicles and your anus becomes one of the strongest parts of your body. I found myself learning how to draw my *prana*, or yogic energy, up through my corporeal center from my nuts. It made all the difference. I may not have been fucking in the lotus position, but when you've got the *mulabahnda* going on, your orgasms are twice, maybe three times longer and more intense. You can't buy that at the pharmacy.

Still, despite those modest improvements, yoga's main sexual accomplishment involved changes to my *attitude*. Since the moment I first sprouted pubes, I'd thought of nothing but sex. It had possessed me like a rampaging demon that could only be briefly exorcised in messy intervals. Sexual desire led me to do a lot of stupid things: I hung around in bars long after I should have gone home, made weird, obsessive phone calls, had naughty exchanges with strangers in Internet chat rooms, and, more often than not, found myself pining, miserable, and frustrated.

As with everything else yoga-related, this astonishing change had philosophical underpinnings. The *Yoga Sutras,* yoga's urtext (which at that point, I hadn't yet studied), understood me perfectly. According to the *Sutras,* all human suffering stems from something called, in Sanskrit, *avidya,* or misperception of the true nature of reality. Suffering clouds the "lens" of the mind and keeps us from seeing clearly. And few things cause more suffering than sex. Just ask Othello, or any human being ever.

Hence the most unpopular of all the sutras, chapter two, verse thirty-eight, which explains the concept of *brahmacharya*. This sometimes gets translated to horrified listeners as "celibacy," meaning that the true student of yoga must be celibate to practice properly. Fortunately, T. K. V. Desikachar, the wisest living scholar of the *Sutras,* explains it this way in his book *The Heart of Yoga*:

"At its best, moderation produces the highest individual vitality."

In other words: Have sex, sure, but stop seeing it as a game, or a goal. Avoid obsession. Go about your sexual business ethically, causing as little harm to others as possible. Amazingly, as I practiced more physical yoga I felt this happen to me as a palpable mental change. Here I was, surrounded by more attractive, cool, smart, skimpily dressed women than any other time in my life, and I barely felt a tug toward bad behavior. Not only had I learned to control myself, the idea of controlling myself came almost naturally. I realized that I no longer needed sex. Yoga had calmed my inner pervert.

Of course, I learned, the physical aspects of sex don't go away when you practice yoga. When you're sitting sweaty in your basement in your stretchy yoga shorts all day, certain sensations will inevitably arise. I'm no eunuch. But after a while, though I still found sex infinitely pleasurable, I didn't *desire* it any more than three or four times a day, down from a record high of about forty-

five. Learning the tools to control desire, as I lurched into
middle age and therefore probably would have substantially fewer opportunities for sex anyway, made my life a
lot easier.

That said, perhaps I began to like my new yoga body a
little too much. One night, as Regina lay in bed, obviously
ready to put in the mouth guard and lower the eyeshade, I
stood on my side of the bed, naked, twirling my arms and
grinding my hips.

"What are you doing?" she asked.

"I'm showing off my sexy yoga dance," I said.

"That's funny," she said. "I thought you were looking at
yourself in the mirror and farting into the fan."

"Just a coincidence," I said. "You should be admiring
my ass."

"Your ass is very nice, dear."

"I appreciate that."

I continued my dance. Regina got out from under the
covers and sat on her knees.

"Damn, man," she said. "Look at those guns!"

I flexed one of my arm howitzers.

"Namaste, motherfucker!" I said.

"What the hell does that mean?" she said.

"It's my yoga catchphrase."

"You can't have a yoga catchphrase."

"Why not?"

"Because yogis don't have catchphrases. Also, it's totally
obnoxious."

"Whatever," I said. "I can feel the yoga power growing
inside me."

"You idiot," she said.

"Oh yeah?" I said, as I moved toward her amorously. "Can idiots do *this*?"

"Whatever you're going to do," she said, "will have to wait until tomorrow, because I'm very sleepy right now."

"Not a problem," I said. "I can always just masturbate."

"Very romantic, dear."

Regina may have occasionally regretted starting me on the way of the peaceful warrior. But her regret was only at level one, maybe level one/two. Most of the time, I think she enjoyed the yoga version of me.

It was the summer of 2008, and my world had narrowed to a one-mile radius. Either I walked five blocks west to Karuna Yoga, or three blocks north to Mara's house. Regina started getting phone calls and emails from friends: "I saw Neal on St. George, and he was wearing his yoga clothes. At eight in the morning." Regina could only respond, "Yep, that's Neal." I was now that guy with the beard and the hairy legs eternally walking around Los Feliz with the yoga mat slung over his shoulder.

Unless I picked up Elijah from school, I only left the house to do yoga or go to Dodger games. My social life, which once had taken place almost exclusively in dingy bars and rock clubs, had migrated to the early daylight hours I'd been sleeping through for years. Most of the friends I'd made either worked as yoga teachers or practiced seriously. I often had thoughts like, *You know, if I leave now, I could make it to Karuna in time for that restorative class.*

The fact that I *liked* things this way frightened me. I'd heard that yoga was supposed to transform you, but was it supposed to transform you into a guy who only wears sleeveless shirts? Regina started calling me a "stinky yoga hippie," and I couldn't really argue, especially because she meant it as a compliment. I was nicer and calmer and more supportive than I'd been since she'd known me. Yoga had made me feel better, and if I felt better, the family was happier.

One morning in Patty's class, I kicked up smoothly into a handstand against the wall. I tightened my core and lifted through my *bandhas.* My legs floated free for a few seconds. A fellow student, who hadn't seen me practice in a while, said, "Nice work, Neal!"

"I know," Patty said, half-sarcastically. "He's Mr. Yoga now."

Technically, "Mr. Yoga" is the trademarked professional name of Daniel Zatar (pronounced "star") Lacerda, an "ambassador" for Lululemon athletic wear and Nike Endurance Sports. He's the founder of the Zen Yoga Wellness Program, the author of the book *Journey into Anti-Aging Power,* and he once led more than twenty-two hundred people in a round of his board game Yoga Pretzel in an attempt to break the Guinness World Record for the largest recorded game of Twister. I couldn't hold a devotional candle to such a fine yoga résumé, but I appreciated Patty's semi-ironic compliment anyway.

My body was developing nicely, but, more important, yoga had completely taken over my mind, like the bugs that crawl into Chekov's and Paul Winfield's ears in *The Wrath of Khan.* After my morning Ashtanga practice, I'd sit in my basement dazed and exhausted, feeling the sweat crystalize into salt on my forehead. I couldn't do anything for hours but ponder the ceiling popcorn and fiddle with my fantasy baseball roster. On Fridays, after Mara's particularly rigorous practice, I couldn't do anything at all.

I went from class to class in a yogic fog, thinking things like "it's all good. These aren't real troubles. We're part of a higher consciousness and our physical reality is fleeting." It's not that the world's problems didn't bother me, or that I didn't have opinions. Rather than worry about them, though, I merely acknowledged their existence and moved on to the next moment. I was used to ironic detachment, but this was the beginning of *actual* detachment, without irony.

Regina and I started referring this new state of mental being as my "yoga brain," something that she, no longer doing yoga, was failing to achieve. Nothing perturbed me. So when Regina would come downstairs, panicked about something she'd seen on the Huffington Post, I responded with equanimity.

"Sarah Palin said something crazy today!"

"Yes, and it will mean nothing tomorrow. It'll all work out for the best."

"Oh my God, the economy is collapsing!"

"Economies rise and fall. Such is the way of humankind."

"All this smoke in the air is making it hard for me to breathe!"

"Eventually, the smoke will go away."

"The polar ice caps are melting at twenty times the rate predicted just six months ago!"

"Does that really surprise you?"

"I just accidentally knocked the DVR remote onto the floor, and I think it's broken!"

"Goddamn it! Do you know how much those things cost? Now what are we going to do? We're totally fucked!"

My yoga brain didn't extend to everything. I had so much further to evolve. Really, I was just hanging around on the outskirts of yoga culture, like a toddler dipping his toes in the water. I had no idea that someone was about to throw me in without floaties.

4

A Different Kind of Fun

If contemporary Los Angeles was Paris in the '20s for yoga culture, then it was Paris in the '40s for weed, with the Vichy government completely subservient to the power of the herbal *Anschluss*. By 2009, there were more marijuana dispensaries in L.A. than there were Starbucks, and it was easier and cheaper to get dope than it was to renew your driver's license.

About a year after I moved to town, a friend, who I think had gotten tired of me calling him at work to ask if he had any weed, gave me a tip. "You should go see my doctor," he said, "and get a prescription."

"But I can't get a prescription, I said. "I'm not sick."

"Sure you are," he said. "Everyone's sick."

"What do I tell him?"

"Dude. Tell him anything. He doesn't care."

Until that moment, it hadn't occurred to me that I could be a medical marijuana patient. Medical marijuana was for people with AIDS or glaucoma, for those dying in hospices, for old ladies with mouth-foaming dementia. Sure, I had high triglycerides and my jaw muscles sometimes cramped when I yawned too wide, but those just weren't on the same level.

Nevertheless, the next day I found myself driving to a tony office building in Beverly Hills for my appointment with a medical marijuana doctor. Once I'd grasped the concept of limitless weed available in stores, I'd made my appointment pretty quickly.

The office's reception area lacked a receptionist. It was just an empty desk and a rubber plant. The doctor emerged from the other room, six feet tall and super fit. He had sandy blond hair parted in the middle, breath-strip-white teeth, and the tan of a man who doesn't work long hours.

We went into his office, which was two chairs, an empty bookshelf, and a few framed degrees on the wall.

"A friend of mine referred me," I said, and then I gave the friend's name.

The doctor scratched his chin thoughtfully. "I think I might remember him," he said. "I have so many patients."

"Right," I said. "So what did you do before you started doing this?"

"Mostly surf."

There was a brief, uncomfortable silence.

"So tell me why you're here," he said.

I took a breath.

"I've been on antidepressants for several years, and they're not working anymore. Marijuana is the only thing that makes me feel better. You know, it's not like I . . ."

"I believe you," he said.

Well, that was easy! Within five minutes I'd written the doctor a $150 check. He'd signed my medical marijuana permission and stamped it with his green cross-shaped seal. It was good for twelve months.

"Recommend vaporizer & edible," he wrote.

"Cool," I said.

"You should send me your medical records eventually," he said, "but there's no rush."

Thusly licensed and now fully complicit in a system that had begun with good intentions but was now leading California into a downward spiral of crime and environmental degradation, I started hitting the dispensary circuit. I bought from AIDS activists, Russian mobsters, skanky hipsters, a strange cadre of Rastas who operated a "temple" behind the Burrito King, and a bunch of weirdoes who, when I walked in, would hit a gong and yell, "THE PATIENT HAS ARRIVED!!!" These places opened and closed with alarming frequency, so, in the yogic tradition, I learned to not grow attached. When one went down, another three sprung up in its place, as though dispensaries were actually mutating to survive. And if I didn't feel like leaving home, there was always the guy from the "artist's collective" who would bring a suitcase full of awesome strains by my house. Plus, I befriended a couple of growers. After an adulthood lifetime of smoking whatever schwag my friends had at the bottom of their sock drawers, I'd finally gotten the hookup.

But my yoga doctor had a totally different prescription for me.

One day, there was a flier on Mara's coffee table for something called "Yogathon '08."

"What's this?" I asked.

"A bunch of really committed yogis are doing yoga for twenty-four straight hours," she said. "You get to choose your own charity, and then people make pledges."

"That sounds good," I said.

"You should do it, man," she said.

"Me?"

"Why not?"

"I'm not experienced."

"Other people are doing it who aren't that experienced."

"You realize this is like inviting a vampire in for dinner," I said.

"I do," she said.

I thought back to my training at ImprovOlympic (now known as iO Chicago) in the mid–90s, when the world was young and I was at the very bottom of a deep comedy barrel. The late improv guru Del Close had taught me—when he wasn't yelling at me to "stop the scene right now, you god-damn moron!"—that you should always say "yes, and" to any situation. While I completely flopped at improv, I tried to take that philosophy into the world: If someone offers you something even a little bit interesting, never turn it down. Getting invited to do twenty-four consecutive hours of yoga seemed like an ideal "yes, and" scenario. Plus, I didn't have anything else going on that weekend.

"Let me ask my wife," I said.

I went home.

"Hey," I said. "Can I do a twenty-four-hour Yogathon with Mara and some of her friends?"

Regina said: "Oh my God, Neal, are you fucking kidding me?"

"No," I said. "It's for charity."

"What charity?"

"I get to pick."

"What are you going to pick?"

"I don't know yet."

"Are you going to be eating?" she asked. "You get really grumpy when you don't eat."

"Let me check," I said.

When I went to my email, I already had a message from Mara with Yogathon information assuring me that there would be three full meals, and snacks throughout the 24 hours. Also, she informed me the Yogathon would start at 2 AM the Sunday before Labor Day, because "that was the most convenient time for everybody."

I went upstairs to Regina.

"She said there will be meals and snacks," I said.

"Do you really want to do this?" she said.

"I'll train really hard," I said.

"Better you than me," she said.

"It starts at 2 AM."

"Good Lord, dude."

By signing up for the Yogathon I'd accidentally committed an act of *seva*, a key concept in the practice of yoga. The full definition of *seva* varies according to the interpreter. It happens to be the name of a delicious Indian snack food made by deep-frying strands of chickpea flour dough flavored with chili powder, salt, and sometimes coriander. But for yoga purposes, it's the Sanskrit word for "service," comparing well with the Hebrew phrase *tikkun olam*, meaning to "repair the world" through acts of kindness. *Seva* is key to a yogi's continual evolution. Some people teach yoga to homeless teenagers, or the disabled, or offer free community classes in yoga-underserved neighborhoods. My teacher Patty helps build schools in Mexico.

Yoga activist Seane Corn, whose *seva* ranges from the highly bourgeois (running a yoga "oasis" with Arianna Huffington at the Democratic National Convention) to the gritty (teaching yoga to AIDS patients in Africa), had this to say in an interview that I read in *Whole Life* magazine one day while waiting for a class to start: "We take our yoga practice off the mat and bring it out into the world where it really does matter. Because maybe this yoga community is way more powerful than we ever imagined it. I believe this community is going to be responsible for changing the world. As we change ourselves, we create a dialogue within our household that is more inclusive, more accepting, more empowered, and more loving. "

That sounded nice and all, but first I had to choose a charity. I considered Tierra Miguel, a Community Supported Agriculture farm from which we got a box of fresh fruits and vegetables twice a month. This meant that I spent most of the winter with a refrigerator full of turnips. I thought: *Doing a Yogathon to support an organic farm co-operative? Why don't I just grow a ponytail and start calling myself Lord Shiva?*

Then I remembered Elijah's Very Special Charter School. This was, technically, a public school, but it had been waging an extensive capital campaign to build a permanent home atop a former ceramics factory behind the Toys "R" Us in Atwater Village. Later, after that fell through, our focus shifted to a run-down former Salvation Army home for unwed mothers, which also fell through, thank God. We finally settled on a spot in an industrial park, formerly occupied by an ad agency, next to a porn-video warehouse. Obviously, the school had real estate concerns, and Regina and I were on the hook for twenty-six hundred bucks. We didn't actually have the money, which took most of the mystery out of my charity decision. I would do yoga for the school.

They posted my bio on the Yogathon website. My yoga credentials were pretty slim, so I'd sent them this:

"Neal Pollack has taken a bunch of yoga classes here and there. Though he still considers himself a beginner, he has perfected the rare and difficult foot-in-mouth position . . ."

This photo accompanied my biography.

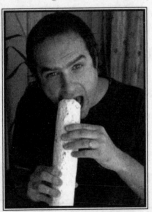

I sent out a donation request letter to friends and family:

I'll be doing twenty-four consecutive hours of yoga from 2 AM on August 31 until 2 AM on September 1. In case you were concerned, the organizers inform me that will be meal breaks, and that

I will also be allowed to use the bathroom whenever I want. The latter will be important, because I don't want the other yogis to see me vomit when I hit the wall. You'll also be invited to the memorial service that will inevitably follow, as I've never done more than two continuous hours of yoga in my life.

A friend went to the website, checked out my bio, and wrote to me, "What the hell are you eating in that picture?"

"A very large Molinari sausage," I replied. "You can buy them at Costco."

"You are dead in this thing," she wrote back. "The sausage is going to come out of your ass halfway through."

But she didn't understand that whim had quickly become obsession. Nothing could stop me. I wanted to do good things; I wanted to be *better.* My best self was peeking over the horizon. I started training, doing yoga nearly every day. The sausage would *not* come out of my ass.

One Wednesday, as I was leaving Ashtanga practice, Mara said to me,

"You're remembering the sequence really well."

"It's amazing, considering I'm stoned 50 percent of the time," I replied.

"I don't want to know that," she said.

"Oh, never in the mornings," I said.

Before coming to practice that morning I'd taken several nice long puffs off the vaporizer. She could probably tell that I was lying, or at least I thought she could. Yoga doesn't entirely get rid of weed-related paranoia.

The next Friday, my paranoia was made manifest as I took a led Ashtanga class with two other students. One was

Mara's Yogathon co-organizer, a very kind, smart, even-keeled blonde who, in the business world, went by the name Linda Richards, but when she taught *Kundalini* yoga, which she'd been doing on and off for many years, she called herself Prabhu Prakash, a name given to her by the Yogi Bhajan himself. The other student in the class was Patty, my regular teacher. I felt like a freshman that had accidentally wandered into a senior seminar.

Mara sat cross-legged on a pillow at the front of the room. As she usually did before Friday class, she gave a little talk. It went like this:

"Patthabi Jois, the founder of Ashtanga Yoga, says that mankind's pleasure-seeking ways are a disease that affect body, mind, and spirit."

Oh boy. This was going to be a real party.

"And like any disease, people display symptoms. They can be emotional symptoms, like anger, sadness, or fear, or they can be physical, in the form of rashes, headaches, and stomach problems. Most of all, it leads to confusion of the mind. Only through yoga can you achieve true bliss and charity and find another way of pleasure. A different kind of fun."

Considering the other people in the room, I felt pretty certain these comments were directed at me. Mara was, not all that subtly, trying to help me get beyond the exhausting veneer of physical yoga. She had spot-on timing. As my yoga brain developed, I'd begun to suspect that something deeper and stranger lay out there beyond the perfect *asana*. I felt hints of something big in the universe that I couldn't quite grasp; the edges of my personality were beginning to soften and ease into calm and humility. This potential evolution of my consciousness frightened me. It simply didn't fit into the excellent personality I'd spent many hard years constructing. I planned to throw up absolutely every cynical defense I knew.

She was right, though. I definitely fell prey to "mankind's pleasure-seeking ways." Pleasure was good, I thought. I liked pleasure, and what was wrong with that? Los Angeles could be a cruel, hard, friendless place. Two things made it tolerable for me: Yoga and marijuana. They may seem to exist in diametric opposition to each other, but, really, the states of mind brought about by doing yoga and consuming THC aren't really that far apart. Both can alter your perception of mundane reality, both can make you feel gloriously, blissfully alive, and both can cause you to drool on the sofa while watching TV.

After class, I hitched a ride with Patty because I was going to take her class next at Karuna, meaning I'd do tough yoga for three-and-a-half out of four hours. I would rock that Yogathon hard.

"Nice Prius," I said.

"Thanks," she said.

"Is it new?"

"No, it's a 2006."

A brief pause.

"This yoga shit is weird," I said.

"It can be."

"I feel like I'm being drawn into a cult."

"It's a pretty inexpensive cult, as cults go," she said.

That's the sort of argument that wins a guy like me to the cause.

➡

The Yogathon operated on a well-meaning but flimsy business model. If someone wanted to donate, they had to go to the Yogathon website and sign up for their yogi and charity of choice. But then, on a separate page, they had to follow a link to the charity's website and follow more specific donation procedures, as the charities hadn't necessarily been informed of the Yogathon's existence. In other words, there was a vast gulf between the act of pledging and the act of actually donating. I found myself having to talk people through the process.

Many people gave $25 gladly, until they got a response message from the Yogathon that read "we'll keep you in our meditations and our prayers." This caused one comedy-writer friend, for whom language is a blessed sacrament, to write: "now I regret donating." Still, Mom donated generously, and so did dear Aunt Estelle. With only a small amount of effort, I raised $1,300 in less than a month.

I got a call from the parent chair of the fundraising committee at Elijah's school. According to another mother at the school, this woman was the "Ashtanga queen of Hancock Park." While I didn't exactly understand what that meant, I'd obviously chosen the right target for my *seva*.

One day, the Ashtanga queen called me with a financial summary of my philanthropic activities.

"It's just so amazing what you're doing for the school," she said.

"Oh, I don't know about that," I said.

"Seriously, not many people would sacrifice their bodies for their child's education."

"Not a big deal," I said.

I hadn't really thought of the Yogathon in terms of

sacrifice before. This didn't feel like a sacrifice to me. It felt natural and fun. I didn't understand why people were emailing me things like "are you sure you want to do this?" and "you're a lunatic." *Yoga for twenty-four hours,* I thought. *What could be better?*

Clearly, I'd floated pretty far down the yoga river. Now it was time for me to meet my fellow paddlers. The week before the Yogathon, there was a potluck at the home of Linda Richards, otherwise known as Prabhu Prakash. I prepared a tray of hummus and olives, and bought a bag of pita chips at Whole Foods. As I headed out the door, the takeout pizzas arrived, to be eaten by Regina, Elijah, my brother-in-law, and my nieces.

"Oh, man," I said. "I want some of that."

"Sorry, dear," Regina said. "Have fun at your *yoga potluck.*"

"I *am* going to a yoga potluck, aren't I?"

"Yes you are."

One half-hour later, my fellow yogis, yoginis, and I sat cross-legged on pillows at a low-lying table in Prabhu Prakash's living room, otherwise decorated only with a Buddhist altar and iPod player. Most yoga people, I was learning, either live simply on purpose, are always broke, or both. In the far corner was a large Tibetan gong. Besides operating a financial-services consulting company and collecting obscure vinyl, Prabhu (Linda) and her husband James, I soon learned, were also accomplished gong players who actually gave gong concerts and gong workshops.

In addition to Mara, Prabhu, James, and me, the other Yogathoners were as follows: John, heavily tattooed, British, once an Arizona real estate agent, now a chi master;

Stacy, a free spirited foot masseuse who brought a really good bottle of sake; Diana, a tax attorney working on the mysterious "third series" of Ashtanga; Dominic, Diana's husband and/or boyfriend, an elevator-repair technician who specialized in Buddhist meditation; a quiet, mysterious, long-limbed fellow named Andrew; and Lauren, a *kundalini* enthusiast recently relocated from New York City. Not in attendance were Nina, a teacher from Karuna who seemed to think I was funny and sometimes sang in a classical choir, and Hilary, a former improv actress who now specialized in ayurvedic healing and something called "laughter yoga." We were like a yoga-nerd focus group.

I tried to suss out the stoners in the room. In a preparatory email about the Yogathon, Mara had written "if you're going to smoke weed, smoke it outside," which really excited me until I got to the "just kidding" part of the paragraph.

We struggled to find safe conversational ground. Not surprisingly, the first thing we landed upon was our terror of doing yoga for twenty-four consecutive hours. Mara and Prabhu assured us that the Yogathon space had a bedroom off to the side, in case anyone needed to crash for a while. There would also be plenty of blankets and bolsters, and we were free to bring pillows if we wanted.

"People have been known to stay awake for sixty to seventy-two hours with no adverse affects," said John. "Besides, awake is a state of mind, isn't it?"

Easy for you to say, Mr. Chi.

Diana and Dominic rhapsodized for a while about a Tibetan monk they'd just studied with in Vancouver. Then

the women began trading *kombucha* recipes. They univer-
sally agreed that ginger is a good flavoring agent for *kombucha*. Prabhu was growing one, but it was turning out "kind
of gnarly." Stacy said she had some *kombucha* babies to give
away if anyone was interested.

"I fucking hate *kombucha*," I said. "It tastes like Satan's
ass."

John the chi guy laughed, and I knew I'd made a friend.

It was then suggested that we should set up a "confes-
sional camera" in the side bedroom, so we could all express
our private feelings, a la Big Brother.

"Yeah," I said. "Every two hours, one of us will get voted
out of the room."

"We'd better start making alliances now," said John.

"We can call it Last Yogi Standing," said Dominic the
Buddhist elevator repairman.

At least we were all operating from the same reference
base.

About seventy-two hours before the Yogathon, my back
began to hurt in the same place it always hurt. I later learned
that these were muscle spasms around my right sacroiliac
joint, which often gets knocked out of place in the line of
yoga duty. Though I'd get there soon, I hadn't yet reached
the stage of yoga dorkdom where I browsed online through
old *Yoga Journal* articles on how to heal various obscure
joints and ligaments. Instead, I just wanted the pain to split.

I got a tennis ball. Every hour or two, I'd lay down on the
floor of my office for fifteen minutes and roll up and down,
putting pressure in different places, and then I moved on
my side, where I rolled for another fifteen minutes while I

watched the pilot episode of *Mad Men* for the third time. I used the tennis ball in the car and when I took Elijah to that gawdaful *Clone Wars* movie that featured Jabba the Hutt's purple gay uncle.

Sometimes the pain was better than other times, but my healing methods threw the rest of my body out of whack. I started getting pains up and down my back, and in my neck. I swear I strained my right quadriceps. My entire body, it felt, would break down at any minute. I would snap a muscle, pop a disc, blow a tendon, tear a labrum, or crack or pull or strain something really important. I was starting to psych myself out.

"It's OK," Regina said. "It's not a competition. Relax if you need to. No one cares."

"Right," I said. "It's only yoga."

We said this as we lay in bed four hours before the start of Yogathon, watching season one of *Californication*, which we'd rented from Netflix. It was a totally unrealistic show about a low-rent hipster novelist dealing with fading talent and the specter of his waning libido while also trying to maintain a semblance of normal family life in Los Angeles. I swear. Where did they get this stuff?

Afterward, I went into the kitchen to make some strong tea; I was going to get picked up in two hours, and didn't think sleep was on the horizon. My mat was packed, along with my sweat catcher, a towel, deodorant, toothbrush and toothpaste, a change of clothes, and my important notebook for taking notes. Midnight came, and Regina went to sleep.

I went into my basement and did the only thing I could with an hour and a half to kill at midnight—take thirty enormous puffs off my vaporizer. Even with a tolerance like mine, this would keep me good and baked until dawn. I already hadn't slept in seventeen hours, and now I was going to add another twenty-four. Caffeine alone wouldn't do.

The time passed delightfully, because Turner Classic Movies was showing *Silver Streak*. Watching a dated 1970s caper comedy, I decided, is exactly what one should do before going into a yoga immersion. Then I got kind of worried. It was 1:10 AM, and Richard Pryor still hadn't shown up yet in the movie. My ride was coming in twenty minutes. You don't watch *Silver Streak* without seeing Richard Pryor. This augured poorly for the Yogathon. But then he appeared, and, soon after, Gene Wilder was putting on blackface in the train station bathroom. I sat in my basement by myself, screaming with laughter.

Prabhu Prakash and James picked me up at 1:35 AM. I was waiting outside, feeling fresh as a lotus, fortified with Tylenol.

"Who wants to do some fuckin' yoga?" I said.

"Eh heh," said Prabhu Prakash. Her jaw steeled. In the front seat next to her, James looked pale and uncomfortable, like he'd just been released from the TB ward.

"Putting one of these things together is a lot of work," he moaned.

"Well, I'm fucking psyched!" I said.

We drove over to Vermont Avenue to pick up Andrew, who Prabhu Prakash had met at teacher training. She couldn't remember which teacher training, though, as there'd been so many. Anyway, they were friends now.

"He's a yoga *freak*," she said.

Andrew got into the car, looking limber and enthusiastic but a little confused.

"I really wanted to get some sleep before it started, but I couldn't sleep," he said. "So I drank one of those Belgian beers. It tasted so good that I drank another. I think I ended up drinking about four, but I don't remember, because I passed out around midnight."

With that, a third of the people committed to the Yogathon had gathered. One of us was as stressed-out as a wedding planner on game day, another seemed to be dying of pneumonia, a third was drunk, and I was even more stoned than usual. But yoga accepts everyone. As soon as you hit the mat, you're born anew, equal to all other yogis. At least that's what the philosophers say. As I blathered on about what a "fucking great time" we were all about to have, I hoped that the philosophers were right. They may have been, or maybe not. Regardless, our sorry lot drove off to do twenty-four consecutive hours of yoga.

5

Yogathon

The Yogathon took place in a newly built two-story artists' studio, just off I-5, in a light-industrial section of Atwater Village called Frogtown. Judging from the fancy construction and the evident quality of the paintings on the walls, the guy who'd built it was a very successful painter; the palettes alone, spread around on tables like place markers, would have given my painter wife a heart attack of jealousy. The paintings in the room tended modern, toward ironic realism, thereby creating the incongruous situation of doing yoga next to the image of a guy in a lemon-yellow polo-style shirt stabbing his own shadow

with a railroad spike. Every time I went to the kitchen for
a cup of tea, I had to look at a painting of a doll lying in a
coffin with a plastic gun draped over her body.

One aspect of our chosen Yogathon room surprised me.
The floors were made of hard finished concrete. I wondered
if my knees, not to mention my wrists, could handle 24
hours of jumping back into *chataranga*. My joints already
trembled at the thought. At least the surface wasn't gravel.

Other than the fact that our practice floor felt no cozier
than a basement storage area of the Pentagon, I liked the
rest of the room. There were big skylights, but the studio
also seemed to respond well to candlelight. A loft up a metal
staircase featured a bookshelf and rocking chair next to a
drawing table, as though to say, "Julian Schnabel could have
sat here." Fronting the studio was a small two-bedroom
bungalow. The living room's built-in bookshelves contained
every art book, art-history book, and art-theory book ever
written. An adjoining room had a daybed, a carpeted floor,
and a comprehensive bookshelf stocked with the works of
Walter Benjamin, Robert Musil's *The Man Without Quali-
ties,* various Kafka texts, and similar gloomy volumes. Obviously, this wasn't the home of a whimsical man. He was,
however, a generous one, and one of Mara's yoga students.
In gratitude, he gave her painting classes, and now he was
donating space.

We entered the dragon at almost exactly 2 AM. Not everyone had arrived yet, but those who had moved around
quietly, with a mixture of hushed reverence and low-level
fear. I took my measure of the room and set up camp in
the second row of mats. Blankets and other props had been
provided. I folded one and sat down, immediately realizing

that I was really cold because I was sitting in a sleeveless top and shorts in an air-conditioned bunker at two in the morning. Maybe I should have brought a sweatshirt.

By 2:20, a full house of eleven had gathered. Dominic the Buddhist had bowed out at the last second because his elevator-repair job put him on call. Prabhu Prakash sat on a mat at the front of the room. She would lead the first session.

"Has anyone not done *kundalini* before?" she asked.

"Only with you," said Andrew the yoga freak.

I raised my hand.

"Never," I said.

"Are you sure, Neal?"

"I think I'd know," I said.

"Well, just follow along the best you can," she said.

The Sikh Yogi Bhajan brought *Kundalini* yoga, an ancient discipline, to California in the late 1960s. It combines meditation, physical poses, prayer, and breathing exercises. *Kundalini* means "the curl of the lock of the hair of the beloved," a metaphor alluding to the flow of energy and consciousness within each of us. It's also sometimes called "the yoga of awareness" because it awakens the "kundalini," which is the unlimited potential that already exists within every human being, fusing the individual and universal selves into a divine union known as "yoga." When practiced properly, adherents say, *kundalini* raises infinite amounts of potential energy in the body, giving you enhanced intuition, mental clarity, and creative potential, kind of like a pre-Phoenix Jean Grey in *The X-Men*.

I was ignorant of those basic facts while shivering inside that frigid art studio in the middle of the night. All I knew is that Prabhu Prakash opened her mouth and unleashed a deep, soulful sound that turned the room into a vast spiritual echo chamber. Everyone else followed.

"ONNNNNNNNNNNNNNNNNNNNNNNNNNG!" they chanted in unison.

Holy crap, I thought. *I've just joined a cult. And they've got me when my brain is the mushiest.* I needed to steel my ego to prevent breakdown.

"NAAAAAAAAAMO! GURU DEV NAAAAAAAMO!"

A brief pause made me think, well, that could just be a lovely invocation before some yoga. Maybe from here. . .

"ONNNNNNNNNNNNNNNNNNNNNNNNNNG!"

Oh, fuck. There they went again.

"NAAAAAAAAAMO! GURU DEV NAAAAAAAMO!"

They just kept chanting. I found myself feeling a great unease, like when Regina's mother makes me hum carols in church on Christmas Eve, except this involved an ancient language, incense, and much skimpier clothes. Then again, I didn't abandon two nights of sleep so I could stand off to the side and make snarky comments. After about a half-dozen frightening repetitions of the mantra, I joined. I mostly got the sounds right, but found myself thinking, *Who is this mysterious "Guru Dave," and what does he want from me?* This was just enough ironic detachment to keep me from going nuts. If I'd known I was repeatedly chanting: "I call upon the divine wisdom," which is how the mantra loosely translates, I probably would have needed an extra shot of detachment.

After what felt like a very long time, the divine wisdom was sufficiently called upon, the chanting ended, and we proceeded into what I guessed was a normal *kundalini* practice. I've lost memory of many of the exercises to the mists of exhaustion, but I distinctly recall holding each arm in an upturned L shape, like a goalpost, and rotating my body from the waist while blowing out breath rapidly and forcefully. This is known, in some circles, as hyperventilation, but in *kundalini,* it's called the "breath of fire," and it really jacks up your *prana.*

We did much fire breathing, arm twirling, and leg stretching, and then settled, more or less spent, into a cross-legged meditation. I could hear the crickets and the nightbirds and the faint rush of the highway. Candles and moonlight illumined the room. By now, I'd pretty much been up all night, and my head was full of bees. Our first *savasana* loomed, and I needed to kick back.

Prabhu Prakash turned on the CD player. A magnificent, soulful female voice, backed by a chorus of seraphim and their horns, began to chant, calling upon the divine. The recorded voices penetrated every molecule in the room. *This is it,* I thought. *The aliens are coming to get me right now.*

"ONNNNNNNNNNNNNNNNNNNNNNNNNG!" they went. NAAAAAAMO! GURU DEV NAAAAAMO!"

Along with the recording, we chanted, our voices enveloped by the choir, and then we chanted again, and then we chanted for a while more. At this point in the practice, according to *kundalini* enthusiasts, you should feel as though a heavenly white light is emanating from every pore as you connect with the infinite through song. Then the music seemed to fade, until it just got stronger and went on for another five minutes? Ten? Fifteen? Six hours? I could no longer tell.

"ONNNNNNNNNNNNNNNNNNNNNNNNNNG!
NAAAAAAAAAMO! GURU DEV NAAAAAAAAMO!"

Finally, mercifully, the music released us from its ethe-really fascist grip. Prabhu Prakash declared *savasana*. I prepared for a rest deeper than sleep.

Then someone started hitting a gong, either Prabhu or James, I never found out; maybe the gong played itself. This was no Chuck Barris gong. It made a noise at once booming and tinny. Eternal, far-out waves of sound enveloped my body as I lay there wondering if my wife would remember to TiVo *Mad Men* while I was gone. And what about the Dodgers? When would they turn that losing streak around?

With that, rational thought ended. The music cradled me, scooping me off the floor, lifting me somewhere beyond the sea. My mind reached toward the void. I saw an infinite number of bright-yellow stars traveling past me at unclockable speeds. Purple and orange comets streaked past my eyes. Time and dimension lost all meaning. A giant fetus floated into view, grander than all creation, and extended its arms toward me. It looked like the Star Child from *2001*, only wiser and more serene.

Holy crap, was I stoned!

The gong faded. Prabhu Prakash called us back to reality. We sat up again, cross-legged, arms extended across the knees, thumb and forefinger joined in a *mudra*. Our practice would end, she said, with the chanting of the words "Sat Nam." This was Sanskrit for "God's name is truth."

"Join your hands together at your heart," she said, and then bellowed "SAAAAAAAAT."

"SAAAAAAAAT," we all said with her.

"NAM," I said.

No one else said "Nam." I'd come in one beat too early. My voice was the only one in the room. *This,* I thought, *is just like Homer Simpson not knowing when to stop "The Monorail Song."* Hold it, was I really supposed to be thinking about *The Simpsons* during yoga?

"Oops," I said.

"NAAAAAAAAM," everyone else said.

Then it was over. The sun hadn't yet risen. We all got off our mats and started moving around the room like monks at vespers, acknowledging one another's presences with whispers and silent nods. I grabbed a handful of nuts off the snack table and put the teakettle on the stove.

A few minutes later, tea in hand, I examined the "gift bag" that Mara and Prabhu had given us. Nobody does anything in L.A. unless there's some swag involved. Mine included a devotional candle bearing the image of Krishnamacharya, the founder of modern yoga. Also there was a gray "Bodhi Booty" T-shirt depicting an Indian deity playing the sitar with the words WHAT ARE YOU THINKING? underneath. The deity held a card that read, "Seek ye not riches, but seek ye wisdom." At the moment, I wanted to seek something better tasting than the health-food bars they'd included in the bag. The organizers had written me a personal note:

"Dear Neal," it said. "Thank you so much for hopping on board Yogathon '08! We hope all this 'positive vibration' doesn't tarnish your bad boy rep! It's so, so fun to have you in the mix!"

Oh yeah, I thought. *I'm yoga's ultimate bad boy.* Why was everyone being so nice to me?

John the chi guy approached. He extended a bottle of

pills. I interpreted this as a gesture of friendship.

"It's a mild stimulant," he said.

In general, if someone offers me a pill, I take the pill. This isn't a wise policy, but I still follow it. I needed all the stimulants I could take. We still had twenty-two hours to go.

At 7:15 AM, a guest baker and yoga student served us a breakfast of homemade banana nut muffins, scones, and Rice Krispies treats. I ate one of each, and also some pita bread with turkey and havarti cheese, plus a banana, some nuts, a hard-boiled egg, and then another banana. After five consecutive hours of yoga, I was damn hungry.

Since the end of my *kundalini* space trip, I'd done a full *hatha* practice led by Mara, essentially the same thing I did at her house every week, except that it started four hours earlier. Compared with what I'd experienced during the night, this felt like a vigorous session of dawn aerobics, except that my lower back hurt and I eased off certain poses.

"Two hours in and already trouble with forward bend?" Mara said.

Quit nagging me, wouldja? I thought.

"I got it covered," I said.

Eye of the tiger, Pollack.

After that practice ended, it was time to get to know my fellow participants through "partner yoga." We were told to hook up with someone who had our astrological sign. That's how I found myself lying on top of James' back while he hunched his head toward his knees. Soon after, because we'd both once lived in Phoenix, John the chi guy and I were taking turns lifting each other in the air with our feet. I do this with my son all the time when I give him an "airplane," but John weighed five times what my son does. Still, I held him. My *bandhas* were strong.

Next, Mara had John and I move into a position where we touched palms and crossed legs at the calves. She told us to gaze at each other. We giggled nervously, like most straight guys would when frozen together in a pose with homoerotic undertones.

"Heh," I said. "This reminds me of the dance they did in *Top Secret!*"

"Yeah," he said, nodding.

"You know, the one where they bop each other on the head and then kiss on the cheeks and she says my name is Hillary and he says what does that mean and she says . . ."

My voice lowered to a whisper because there was actually someone named Hillary in the room: "*She whose bosoms define gravity* and he said my name's Nick and my dad thought it up while shaving. That one."

"I'm sorry, what?" said John.

"You know. *Top Secret!* The Zucker Brothers movie. From 1984. It's only like the greatest comedy of all time."

"I haven't seen it."

"Shop at Macy's and love me tonight," I said. "Heh."

Seriously, was I really expecting someone to get a *Top Secret!* reference at the Yogathon? As we kept our legs locked and kept gazing at each other for many uncomfortable minutes, happy thoughts of Omar Sharif tottering around encased in a crushed car, of surfers shooting skeet, and of singing horses carried me through.

Mara had a way of sensing when I was descending into unforgivable superficiality. She walked over to us and said:

"One of the many meanings of yoga is focusing your attention on a fixed point for an extended period of time. That focused attention, that intensity of gaze, allows us to think positively with one mind and to transform the world."

There she went again. Of course, she was right. I really did need to focus for a little while. I'd been spending more time at the Yogathon thinking about Manny Ramirez than about transforming the world. Admittedly, Manny, not yet revealed to the world as a big cheater, had been on an unprecedented hot streak for the Dodgers and I was excited. I couldn't help it; my best self loved yoga, but I was also a baseball fan and an aficionado of '80s comedies. Would I remain forever bogged down in my frivolous pleasure-seeking ways? The next eighteen hours would reveal all.

6

Too Many Tibetans

11:30 AM: John leads us through a chi exercise in "strengthening will." In order to generate chi, he says, you must do eight smooth, cool movements eight times each. They are called such things as "Drawing the Bow and Letting the Arrow Fly," "Big Bear Turns from Side to Side," and, my personal favorite, "Punching with Angry Gaze." But after ten consecutive hours of yoga, learning another discipline, even if it's metaphysically related, feels like a lot of work. I rally myself by thinking . about the opening ceremonies of the Olympics and how the Chinese are very disciplined at kicking our collective asses.

The least I can do is eight reps of "Wise Owl Gazes Backward."

After the exercises, using the chi we've built up, John has us craft large imaginary blue balls of energy with our hands. Then we stretch the balls and condense them into tinier balls. True masters, John says, can use chi energy to knock pictures off walls or even break windows with their minds. Amazing. If I could master the chi, I think, then I could teach my son how to use The Force, and then he'd think I was the greatest dad ever.

After the demonstration, I ask John, "Is chi made up of midi-chlorians, tiny particles that surround us, permeating every living thing?"

But he doesn't get the reference.

12:45 PM: All day, I've been watching people wilt and then fall over in the middle of a meditation or even a standing pose, then gently slide into a coma underneath a small pile of blankets. Up to now, I've resisted collapse. Then Diana the Buddhist lawyer fronts a "core integration" *hatha* yoga session. I fully intend to do this all the way through, but about five minutes in, I find myself overwhelmed by a vast wave of nausea and self-loathing even greater than the ones that usually overtake me in the middle of the day. My core is integrating right into itself, like an imploding star. If I don't sleep, I'll die. I stagger out of the studio and into the house, black spots flashing in front of my eyes. Mercifully, the daybed is unoccupied. I pass out. When I open my eyes, only a half hour has gone by, and the core integration hasn't even entered its wind-down phase. I rejoin the practice, proving that, at this point, I can even do yoga in my sleep. I take out my notebook and write, "I've slept maybe an hour in the last thirty-six, and I feel surprisingly alive." I immediately hate myself for writing this.

2 PM: Lunchtime. Patty arrives bearing a tray of sandwiches from Leaf, a raw-food deli in Sherman Oaks. There's also a bowl of something else, distinctly pungent, that she's brought from home. She calls me over to her with a subtle gesture.

"Don't tell anyone," she says, her voice lowering to a whisper. "*It's tuna.*"

4 PM: Stacy pairs us up to give one another foot massages. As a courtesy, people stick their feet in the kitchen sink and scrub down with soap and paper towels. I'm assigned to James, but he and I stare at each other in extreme distaste. We've been getting along fine, but the last thing either of us want to do after fourteen consecutive hours of sleepless yoga is massage another dude's dirty feet. Instead, he gets to massage his wife. They kiss tenderly enough to force me to look away in embarrassment. I'm assigned to Hillary, who, in addition to her many other talents, is a master of yogic massage. She slathers me with creams and unguents. I moan with pleasure like I'm in a homemade porn video, and all she's doing is rubbing my calves.

Then it's my turn. Hillary's leg slips around in my grip like I'm trying to pick up a whole snapper at the fish market. Stacy has to step in and do my work for me. She gives me many tips, none of which register. I start massaging Hillary again.

"How'm I doing?" I ask. "Not very well, right?"

She sighs.

"You're fine, Neal," she says.

Next, Nina is supposed to lead us in a session of *Hatha* Yoga Nurturing Self and World, but everyone's clamoring for a half hour of hand massage instead, including Nina herself. We're told to stay with our partners. Hillary gives me a look of minor warning. "Do the best you can," she says. I do. Afterward, she takes my right hand and squeezes between the thumb and index finger.

"SONOFABITCH!" I yell. "OW! OW! OW!"

"Too much pressure?" she says.

"No, it's just right," I say. "I type a lot."

5:30 PM: I write, "My brain is rotting out my skull. I feel near lobotomized. My legs are throbbing with pain." Obviously, the Yogathon has diminished my prose. Only one thing can freshen my brain. I go into the bathroom with my towel and turn on the shower. Hot water proves elusive. After a few minutes wandering around the stall, I get out without having wet my hair. My mind wanders to the hot shower that awaits me in nine hours at home. Also, the Dodgers are playing the Diamondbacks tonight. I tell myself to focus my attention, like Mara wants, but I find that I'm not listening very well right now.

6:30 PM: Lauren leads us through a session of "liver-cleansing" *kundalini,* and it feels like it's never going to end. I jump around on my mat, flapping my hands, with my elbows by my side. We look like a bunch of goddamn short-bus hippies. Later in the practice, we partner up; I draw Nina. We're told to wrap our feet around each other's hips and our hands around each other's necks and move around in a circle to the beat of some horrific techno *bhangra* Kylie Minogue music. My liver's been cleansed, alright—of dignity. Nina's apparently having the same thought that I am. We look at each other and, at once, tip over onto the floor, howling with laughter.

"I'm so glad you're here," she says.

"Really?" I say. "No one's ever glad that I'm *anywhere*."

"Oh, silly," she says.

8 PM: Dinner arrives in the form of takeout Thai food. There's more than enough for everyone, but I nonetheless appropriate a container of spicy papaya salad, holding it like my dog Shaq when he wraps his paws around that disgusting squeaky rubber newspaper with the picture of Garfield on the front. I know that the salad will give me gas and that the gas will lead to inhuman smells, but I don't care. We're eighteen hours in. I'm going to let them rip.

10 PM: After a long "restorative" yoga session that finds me wrapped in blankets with a bolster shoved up my ass, John leads us through a hypnotherapy session. His sonorous voice goes: "Get comfortable . . . become relaxed . . . take a deep breath . . . hold it . . . close your eyes. . . ." He has us count down backwards from one hundred. By the time I reach ninety-eight, I'm somewhere else. Lord knows what he says to us then, or for how long, but somewhere between ten and forty-five minutes later, I hear, "And you know you have taken a big step forward on your path toward true enlightenment. You are still feeling relaxed and at ease. You are feeling warm and comfortable as you continue to bathe

in the soft glow of the healing, soothing white light."

Wait, I thought. *What white light? No one said anything about a white light!* As far as I know, I've just undergone some sort of New Age assassin's training. I'll be the Manchurian Yogi.

Afterward, we take a short break. Regina has sent me a text message informing me that the Dodgers have beaten the Diamondbacks handily.

"Whoo-hooo!" I say.

"What?" says Diana the Buddhist lawyer.

"Dodgers won," I say.

She sniffs dismissively.

"Now now," Nina says. "It's important to him."

"Thank you, Nina," I say.

Actually, it's beyond important. The team, in the middle of a horrific losing streak, has just beaten the best two starters of their main divisional rivals in a row, on the road. This is how champions are forged, until they lose to the Phillies. How can I focus my attention on anything else?

11:45 AM: Hillary leads us in a session of laughter yoga. We lie on one another's bellies and giggle. There are trust falls. At one point, she says, "Now you need to imagine that you're on the world's most crowded subway." We scrunch together in a ball-like mass and jostle. We're only allowed to speak to one another in gibberish.

"A bloo woo woo woo woo blah blah," I say.

"Echy blechy wechy murgle whoop whoop!" says someone else.

I realize that these are the kinds of highly sophisticated activities we did back at camp Anytown USA. I didn't really like them then, either, but I participated because I loved my fellow campers. Am I doing the same thing here? Is this my best self, running around in a circle, deliberately bouncing myself into strangers while wearing my yoga pajamas? God, I hope not.

1 AM: We chant, in Sanskrit, the *gayatri* mantra, one of the holiest prayers in the world. Then we chant it again, twenty-six more times. Here are the words:

> *OM bhur bhuvah svaha*
> *tat savitur varenyam*
> *bhargo devasya dhimahi*
> *dhiyo yo nah prachodayate*

Translated very simply, it means: "May the Almighty God illuminate our intellect to lead us along the righteous path." It's said that if you repeat this mantra one hundred thousand times, all your wishes will come true. If you say it twenty-seven times, you get one step closer to finishing the Yogathon. I long for a firm mattress and a clean pair of underwear.

"Prabhu Prakash," Mara suddenly declares, "has decided that we need to do the Five Tibetans."

I grit my teeth.

"*What*," I say, "are the Five Tibetans?"

"Oh, nothing too taxing," says Mara. "Just some simple exercises."

The Five Tibetan Rites were first presented to the world in 1939 in a pamphlet called *The Eye of Revelation*, written by an obscure Midwesterner named Peter Kelder. Apparently, Kelder met a "retired British army colonel" while traveling in Southern California. The colonel told Kelder about the exercises, which he'd learned in Tibet and which had restored him to youthful vigor. This sounds very fishy, of course, but yoga contains a lot of vague origin stories. Patthabi Jois, the creator of Ashtanga yoga, for instance, claims that the original Ashtanga sequences, written on leaves, were "eaten by ants," so the core devotional movements of modern Buddhism might very well be the lunatic vision of a drunken crank as told to a schizophrenic snake-oil salesman from Indiana. Or not.

At that moment, after doing yoga in an art studio for twenty-three consecutive hours, I lean toward the latter, especially because the first Tibetan rite is "Clockwise Whirling," with arms extended.

Mara demonstrates.

"And now you do it twenty-one times," she says.

"You've got to be kidding," I say.

But she isn't, and then everyone's whipping around like Lynda Carter circa 1976. I make it through about four rotations before I fall to my mat, gasping. My stomach is now the only thing spinning around, and it's full of Pad Thai. I crawl toward a bolster and drop my forehead.

"OHHHHHHH," I say. "FUUUUUUUCK."

The rites continue, with head and leg raises followed by twenty-one camel poses and twenty-one tabletop poses. Shivering, I squat on my mat. I have a bushy, unkempt beard. My eyes are red and cracked. I wear a blue-and-white yoga blanket around my shoulders. I look like Charles Manson.

Yet when it comes time for the fifth Tibetan, which involves jumping back into downward dog twenty-one consecutive times, I rally and play along with the group.

"What the hell," I say. "I've come this far."

"That's the spirit," Mara says, as though she did this every day. Maybe she does.

1:30 AM: The Five Tibetans end. It's time for group sharing. Hillary reads aphorisms off refrigerator magnets. Diana shares six very long chants that she does before her daily Ashtanga practice because, you know, we really need to hear *more* chanting at that point. I'm so tired that everyone might as well be speaking in Urdu.

Merely by participating in this Yogathon, says Prabhu Prakash, we've sent an infinite amount of positive light into the universe. Our actions and generosity on this day have made the world a better place. Yes, I think. This is what I wanted. I'm a better version of myself just for showing up. I've pushed my thirty-eight-year-old body to the brink of disintegration and I've survived. Plus, I did it to raise money for a school. I did it for *the children*. No matter how bad I feel, I still feel good. My best self might actually behave this way, though it would probably remember to wear more deodorant. It truly has been a different kind of fun.

1:45 AM: Hands joined, we sit in a circle swaying back and forth, chanting in Sanskrit. I'm thinking, *it's almost over, it's almost over, it's almost over.*

"After we finish," Prabhu Prakash says, "there will be celebratory dancing."

The group murmurs unenthusiastically.

But first, she says, we have to chant some more. Loosely

translated, the chant goes, "I call upon the divine to keep my brain from leaking out my ears during the night, and that when I wake up, it won't feel like there are bugs crawling under my skin anymore. OM."

2 AM: The Yogathon ends. Prabhu Prakash turns on her "celebratory dancing" music. It's too low-key for this crowd, which would need three tabs of ecstasy and the world's greatest DJ even to consider dancing at this point. She and Hillary stand up and sway from side to side a couple of times. The rest of us almost kill one another running for the light switch. We quietly celebrate by throwing away our trash, rolling up our mats, and getting the hell out of there.

12 PM: After nine hours of sleep, I surprise everyone, including myself, when I'm able to walk upright and carry on a conversation, even though the only thing I want to talk about is yoga. We go to a Labor Day barbecue at my cousin's. The world appears gauzy and pixilated, as though I can see past its mundane, frustrating façade, yet it's also exactly the same as it was before, which is kind of a relief. Really, I don't know how I'm supposed to feel after a Yogathon. Then, after a couple of turkey burgers, my pre-Yogathon digestive system asserts itself and my brain snaps back to normal.

I'm not going to even think about doing yoga again until at least Wednesday.

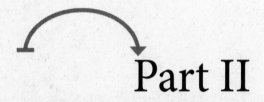

Part II

Rise Out of the Bayou of Your Pelvis

7

Somebody Seva Me

"One of the problems with capitalist yoga," Mara was saying, "is that they have to keep people coming back to class. So they tell you that yoga will save your life. But that's not true. You save your own life."

Every Friday at 8 AM, before leading us through another brutal Ashtanga primary series, she gave a talk along these lines. This week, my mind did a very non-yogic ballet, anticipating the moment later that morning when I was no longer practicing yoga and would be sitting in my basement updating my Facebook profile. So I missed the larger meaning of what

Mara was saying. Save my own life, yeah, yeah. But I did get one meditative thought out of it: Man, she's right. Yoga is fucking *expensive*.

A few minutes after class, I peeled myself off the floor and attempted to engage my teacher in coherent conversation.

"So does your critique of capitalist yoga mean you're going to start giving away classes?" I asked.

"You wish," she said.

Darn right I wished! I was shuttling $100 a month to Mara. That was a great deal for twelve classes of almost totally individualized instruction; elsewhere, I could maybe get one private lesson for that amount. But it was still $100 a month. I had to find a way to cut my yoga costs. Fortunately, though Mara continued to charge me, I discovered a way to take unlimited classes at Karuna Yoga for free.

Karuna managed to stay solvent through a simple system. Volunteers worked one shift a week behind the desk, and were rewarded with unlimited yoga. The studio's owner called this her *seva* program, though there was none of the high-minded talk about universal altruism that you hear from rich West Side yoginis. Here, the "service" was that we helped keep a small neighborhood yoga studio open. That was the kind of altruism I could get behind. After many years of consistent practice at Karuna, I was ready to give back, and, more important, to get back.

I emailed Liz, Karuna's manager, who wrote back quickly, and with more enthusiasm than I'd expected.

"We'd love to have you!" she wrote. "You'll just need to fill out an application (formality) and come in to the studio to train behind the desk. We have permanent shifts opening very soon on Wednesday 6–9:45 PM, and Saturday 4:30–7 PM. Let me know where your interest lies and then we can talk about coming in to train!"

The Wednesday shift seemed kind of long, but I couldn't see myself getting three hours every Saturday afternoon from my wife. So I told Liz my interests lay with Wednesday. The next time I was at the studio, I filled out a formality application.

"Let's do the training next Monday," I later emailed Liz. "Late morning, early PM would be best for me."

She wrote back: "I'm only at the studio 8:30 to noon on Mondays, but right now I'm available next Wednesday evening, so maybe we can just do the whole shift together? That might be best anyway, so you'll be able to get the whole run of the day with closing."

As I soon learned, these were the sorts of negotiations that comprised the *seva* system. A lot of the *sevas* were actors or musicians or low-level film industry workers. Last-minute shoots or auditions would force them to get other *sevas* to cover their shifts, and then the cover people would have something come up and they'd need someone to cover for them. Half the time, when my cell phone rang, it was a breathless yoga freak trying to get me to take a shift. The other half, it was my wife.

But the most important point had yet to be nailed down.

"Can I start taking free classes yet?" I wrote.

"I'll go ahead and put you in the computer as a *seva* unlimited so you can come on in!" Liz wrote back.

"Thanks!" I said. "Oh, also, I'm not in town next week, so I already have to miss my first shift."

"No problem," she wrote back. "I'm filling in for you. The owner is very excited to have you, and so am I!"

I was really going to like this *seva* business.

Eventually, on some other Wednesday evening, I got around to my training. I discovered many things about Karuna Yoga that I hadn't known before. Before that night, I'd paid no attention to anything behind the sheer gold curtain. My training was like learning how the yoga sausage gets made.

For example, I learned that Karuna's owner liked the floor to be shiny when she came in at dawn to teach the first class of the day. The person who closed the studio the night before achieved this shininess by running a dry Swiffer over the studio floors, followed by a wet Swiffer. The owner preferred a particular Swiffering motion, basically a figure eight with an extra half-loop at the end. She could always tell the next morning if the *seva* had gotten lazy and done a straight Swiff instead. So, really, it was better to Swiff the way she wanted. Though I never got reprimanded for bad Swiffering, and hadn't heard of that happening to anyone else, I wasn't interested in becoming a cautionary *seva* tale.

There was a tiny iPod Shuffle that remained on at all times, even overnight, because the owner wanted the sound of a mantra continually playing in the studio. However, the iPod Shuffle lost its power quickly, so it needed to be charged at all times behind the desk during class, usually while I was dealing with the class check-in system, which operated on a nightmare Windows software program called FileMaker Pro. It had many obscure aspects, many of which needed to be explained in cute little notes taped to the monitor. A simple request, like when a teacher wanted to bring a guest to class, required at least ten data-processing steps. After years of relying on Gmail and Google Documents, I felt like I was suddenly being forced to work at the vehicle-registration bureau in Soviet-era Poland. It made me nervous.

Each *seva's* shift also carried a special "task." These included watering the plants, cleaning the mouse and keyboard, and restocking the paper towels. I drew a real lemon: cleaning all the rental mats, on both sides, with either Clorox Disinfecting Wipes or Simple Green cleaner and paper towels. I'd have to do this every week. At first I thought it was a kind of hazing ritual for newbies, but it turned out that I just had gotten unlucky.

"Oh, great," I said.

"It's not so bad," said Liz. "Just be sure to do it in a figure eight motion."

I couldn't tell if she was being wry or not. But I got a bead on her quickly. We spent the rest of the evening sharing a chocolate bar and browsing various humor websites, including The Best of Craigslist and one that sold ironic greeting cards. The next night, I was watching Comedy Central and saw her on an old episode of *Chappelle's Show,* where she played a woman who wished she had really big boobs, and then some Chappelle-style fairy gave her the wish. Soon, she started showing up on my TV all the time. Only in L.A. can your yoga supervisor also be the girl from the Vonage commercial.

The next week, I had my first solo shift. I put eye pillows by the door for the teacher because I remembered she'd used them the week before, and I made sure to have the exact right number. The teacher looked at me, astonished.

"How did you know?" she said.

"*I remembered, I remembered,*" I said, in the voice of a little child.

"You're an all-star *seva* for sure," she said.

One week, and I'd already made the all-star team.

Afterward, Liz called me.

"I just wanted to make sure everything went OK," she said.

"I didn't burn the studio down," I said.

"Good for you," she replied. "Do you want a cookie?"

Soon, I developed a *seva* routine. Five minutes before my shift was supposed to start, I pulled my 1998 Nissan Sentra into my assigned parking place behind the building, smoked a hefty bowl of weed, got out, and unlocked the studio. I checked the lights and thermostat, stood behind the welcome desk, and waited for people to appear. Then they did, and then they did yoga. Ten minutes after class started, it was my job to peek in and ensure that the number of students in the class equaled the number on the sign-in sheet. Since there were often only five or six students on the sheet, it was hard to ever miss anyone, but I had to follow protocol nonetheless.

Then I went outside and organized all the students' shoes into orderly rows. This wasn't required, but Liz said the students really thought it was marvelous. I wondered if this was true or if it was just some obsessive tic of hers; usually, when students came out of class, they were so blissfully worked-over that they wouldn't have cared if their shoes were hanging above them on an electrical wire. But it did look nice, so I performed my duty.

Once the last class was over, I took out the trash, closed

the curtains and the bathroom window, and cleaned the mats. This task (which was later, mercifully, replaced by the easier job of cleaning the bathroom mirrors with Windex) proved as disgusting as it sounded. The mats got cleaned three times a week or so, but I had no way of knowing which ones had been used in that time, or how often, so I had to subject them to a smell test. The ones that smelled damp and salty, I cleaned. The others, I left. Sometimes, though, I'd feel guilty, and I'd resniff the mats I hadn't cleaned, determining that they did, in fact, need to be cleaned. My nose became attuned to the different levels of sweaty glaze on yoga mats. God, I hated that part of the job.

I spent the rest of my time managing my fantasy baseball team, checking email, and wondering why the apartment across the alley had sixteen Thai women inside. They were gone by the time the shift ended, so I knew they didn't live there. Mostly, they seemed to spend their time shelling peas and watching TV. Occasionally, Chassidic Jews would come and go. In a big city, it's usually better to not ask questions.

One night everything was going great until the first two customers walked in and wanted to buy class passes.

"We're interested in the strength and the stretching," one of them said.

You poor suckers, I felt like saying to them. I used to want the strength and the stretching, too, but now I want more and more. Yoga is the roach motel of activities. You can check in, but you can never check out. You think it's a cure, but it's really a sickness. This is going to eat your soul.

"You'll get that here," I said.

"Because we came before, and it was a lot of breathing."

"That was probably a *kundalini* class," I said.

The first girl handed me her debit card. I swiped it three times, but it didn't take. I turned it the other way and it worked. Now I couldn't figure out how to enter a new invoice on the computer. Meanwhile, other students had signed in, ten minutes had passed, and I still had another debit transaction to do.

"Um, Amber?" I said to the evening's teacher, who had once been a *seva*. She was next to me fiddling with the eye pillows. "How do you create a new invoice?"

She did that for me, but then I had to do *another* credit card transaction. This filled me with fresh panic. *Maybe I shouldn't get stoned before my shift*, I thought, and then I thought, *nah, I'd be just as bad at this regardless, and then I wouldn't be stoned*.

"That's $125," I said.

"Isn't the new-student pass $100?" said the guy.

"Oh, right."

I feared something would go horribly wrong on my watch: The incense would start a fire. A plant would fall over. I'd drop the owner's iPod or spill water on the computer. Maybe I'd accidentally charge a student $600 or lose a receipt.

This was why I'd tried to avoid actual work my entire life. Any time I'd had a job other than writing, I'd been fired within three months. The only exception was the time after high school when I worked for a bankrupt novelty store in Scottsdale whose owner was dying of cancer and therefore had other problems besides my incompetence. I was sure that eventually Karuna's owner was going to fire me. From a volunteer job.

➡

The *seva* gig worked great for me until the Dodgers traded for Manny Ramirez, which threw my entire autumn into question.

At around 8:45 PM one Wednesday in September, I was sitting in the yoga studio, waiting for Tanya's class to end so I could clean the mats and go home and watch the rest of the Dodgers game. The fading Diamondbacks had already lost humiliatingly to the Cardinals, again, knocking the Dodgers' magic number down to two, meaning the team was about to clinch a division title. Now the Dodgers had the bases loaded against the Padres, who by the end of the season were fielding a Triple-A club, and not even a very good one. My friend Jerod called.

"I'm listening in the car," he said. "Are you watching?"

"I'm watching on ESPN GameCast," I said.

"Why are you whispering?"

"Because it's the night I volunteer at the yoga studio."

"You're watching the game at the yoga studio?"

"If I volunteer, I get free classes."

"That's classic. So do you know what's going on?"

"The computer is a little slow."

"Well, they just yanked Estes, and Manny's coming up."

"Hang on, I'm gonna go outside."

I did, and then I could stop italicizing my voice.

"FUCK, DUDE!" I said. "THEY'RE GONNA FUCK-ING DO IT! THIS HAS BEEN THE MOST AWESOME MONTH EVER!"

"I know, right?"

"We've gotta start planning for the playoffs!"

"Totally," he said. "Let's talk tomorrow."

I went back into the studio. Manny grounded out to second during *savasana*. But he homered later as part of a six-run eighth inning, and the Dodgers went on to dismantle the Padres 12–4. Jerod sent me a text message, which I received while wet-Swiffing the studio floor.

"Manny!" It read. "53 RBI in 50 games with dodgers."

Jerod and I were united in our belief that the Dodgers would make a miracle run to the title. Over the next week, we spent many minutes on the phone and online trying to figure our budgets and our time so we could attend as many Dodger playoff games as possible, or at least watch them on TV in full, live, without the aid of TiVo. It was like when I was eleven years old and miraculously got very sick in the fall of 1981 so I could stay home from school to watch the Dodgers beat the Astros and then the Expos and then the Yankees and then Steve Garvey had champagne all over him.

Major League Baseball released the playoff schedule. The Dodgers drew the Cubs in the first round. They would open the series on a Wednesday, at 3:30 PM. Oh, this was bad. I wouldn't miss my *entire* shift, unless the game went into extra innings, but it still made me curse the day I ever became a *seva*. Baseball fandom is exemplary of what yoga gurus refer to as an "unnecessary attachment." I get the concept; unless you actually play or work for the team in question, their achievements aren't actually yours even though you pay Frank McCourt's extortionate parking fee. You shouldn't allow your emotions about sports teams get in the way of your actual life, your search for a better self. But after Kirk Gibson's 1988 home run to win game one of the World Series, I felt a level of ecstatic transcendence that

I haven't since. I definitely had best-selfness going on that evening, and I wanted it back. This was the *Dodgers*. They meant something to me. Couldn't they be yoga, too?

Immediately, I began to scramble for a sub. I emailed Liz first. She replied:

"October 1 is my thirtieth birthday. Sorry, sucka."

With that avenue closed, I called upon Carly, who I'd swapped with before. On September 28, I sent her a desper-ate email. "I should be able to get there by 7, MAYBE 7:30," I wrote. "But no later than that. So if you subbed, you'd have to check people in for Amber's class, but not do the dirty work of cleaning up the studio and the rental mats and all the other unsavory stuff I do at the end." She said she might be able to help me out, but then wrote me back that she had to help her boyfriend move that day. What was with these selfish people? Didn't they understand that the Dodgers were in the *playoffs*?

The next day I sent out a blanket email to all the *sevas*. It contained the word "PUH-LEEEEEESE," spelled and capi-talized just like that, so they'd know I was desperate. Pretty quickly, two *sevas* got back to me. One of them was the Slavic supermodel that I'd stormed out on two years previ-ous because she'd been giving me unwanted adjustments. Now she was doing something nice for me, and I really felt bad. Because of that, I took the other offer, from a kind-hearted comp-lit graduate student.

That Wednesday, Jerod and I sat down in front of my flat-screen at 3:30 PM to watch the Blue's march toward glory. And when James Loney hit that grand-slam in the top of the fifth, marking the beginning of the Cubs' end, I dropped to my knees, moaning with joy. I got to my shift at 7:15, sweaty, stoned, drunk, and wearing a dirty Dodgers cap. No one noticed or commented. There are few baseball fans in Yoga Land. I immediately began to worry about what I'd do about my shift if the Dodgers made it to the World Series, when the games are all in the evenings. But the Phillies took care of that problem in five.

I could tell Liz had been getting frustrated with the job. The notes taped to the keyboard had been growing more numerous and more desperate-sounding. Perhaps part of the problem was that *sevas* had her cell-phone number and email, and that they weren't afraid to use it. Also, she made herself too available on gchat, so we treated her as though she was constantly on duty. Here's one telling exchange:

Me: Hey! All is well here . . . but I can't find the ligh switch for the main overhead. It's getting dark!
Liz: In the closet behind the water bottle
Me: thanks!

Soon after, she was gone. The studio continued to function. By then, I knew where all the light switches were, and also where to find most of the office and cleaning supplies, though certain things remained unclear to me. Four months after I started, the owner had to show me how to ring up an order when someone bought a yoga mat. The next month, she had to show me how to print out a receipt. Regardless, I became a fixture at the studio, the bearded guy working the desk on Wednesday nights. I developed inside jokes with various students. Gradually, I learned their names and had them registered before they could even make it to the sign-in sheet. One of them asked me,

"So when are you going to start teaching?"

"Heh-heh," I said. "I'm never going to be a yoga teacher."

"Sure you will," she said.

No one who *actually* knew me would have said such a thing. One night, a friend came into the studio. She didn't know I was working the desk. When she saw me standing there with my kind *seva* smile, she laughed semi-evilly.

"*What*?" I asked.

"I can't believe you're the guy handing out yoga mats," she said.

"Why not?"

"Because you're the most selfish person I know."

"I'm not that selfish."

"Yes you are."

"I'm nice!"

"You're nice-ish."

No, dammit, I was more than "nice-ish." I'd begun my transformation into a yogi, a fully aware surfer of reality's highest planes. In fact, during my off minutes behind the *seva* desk, I read the owner's copy of the *Bhagavad Gita*, in the beautiful translation by Steven Mitchell.

The *Gita*, one of the most sacred Hindu texts, originally appeared as a seven-hundred-line section of the *Mahabarata*, one of the two major Sanskrit epics of ancient India. It takes the form of a conversation between Arjuna, a heroic warrior, and his chariot driver (played by Robin Williams), who, on the eve of a great battle, reveals himself to be the incarnation of the great Lord Krishna. In an astonishingly short amount of time, Krishna delineates the four main yogic paths: devotional service, action, meditation, and knowledge. He also says that the ultimate goal of yoga is to detach oneself from the ego and communicate with the universal truth of the divine. However, Krishna also tells Arjuna that it's important to take right action when in your physical form, because otherwise the world would fall into chaos. He then totally blows Arjuna's mind by revealing to him the totality of the cosmos.

While I read it between hands of online poker, the *Gita* profoundly affected my mind. At that moment, I started to practice detaching myself from grief, sorrow, and the relentless buzz of activity that plagues our lives, as well as the fact that some guy from Germany was kicking my ass at Texas hold 'em. I learned about the seven stages of yogic wisdom and began to make a conscious effort to tamp down any outward manifestations of selfhood. Sometimes, I updated my Facebook status to let people know I was doing this.

One afternoon, midway through a substitute *seva* shift, I sat on a stool while baked out of my nuts, idly picking my nose until class got out. A handsome young dude entered. He said that the owner had asked him to drop off a *seva* application, and he handed it to me.

His most recent job had been waiting tables in New York City. *Obviously an actor*, I thought. Then I noticed that he'd once been an editorial assistant at the *Chicago Reader*, where I'd worked for seven years. Since the paper, like all papers, was more or less in the process of financial collapse, this probably wasn't a coincidence that I'd run across many more times in my life.

"The *Reader*, huh?" I said.

"Yeah," he said.

"I used to write for that paper."

"Really?" he said. "What's your name?"

I told him.

Now, when I drop my name to another writer, my expected response is "Oh my God, dude! I totally love your stuff! It's really great to meet you!" Or at least, "Oh yeah, sure. I've heard of you."

He stared at me blankly.

"Maybe I read you in the archives," he said. "I spent a lot of time reading the archives when I worked there."

"So did I," I said.

Suddenly, I felt old, useless, and insecure. I easily had ten years on this guy. All the yoga philosophy in the world couldn't counteract the horrifying feeling of obsolescence that washed over me at that moment. Still, I tried to make conversation. We talked about the death of newspapers, but how long can you do that, really? Eventually, as every conversation in my life did, the topic turned to yoga.

"So do you practice a lot?" I asked.

"Nah," he said. "But I'm working on a pilot about a yoga studio. I figured I should see what one was like."

Rookie mistake, kid. You never know who you're talking to in L.A., or what kind of lunatic ulterior motives they have. For instance, you could be talking to a guy who was working at the same yoga studio, who maybe in the back of his mind harbored fantasies about writing his *own* yoga sitcom. And maybe this guy felt threatened.

"Do you have an agent?" I asked, hoping that my voice would drown out the sound of my sinking heart.

No, he said. But friends were showing his other work around to agents. It probably wouldn't take long.

"Cool," I said.

He left. I took the application into the owner's office. As I sat there, staring at the paper, I felt a Good Krishna hovering over one shoulder and an evil Krishna over the other. Do it, the devil said. This guy is your competition. He's cutting in on your territory. The angel said, come on, man, he's just a kid. Give him a break.

The market for yoga-based entertainment was surprisingly fat. I'd done my research and had seen trailers and pilots for a half-dozen independently produced yoga sitcoms. There was the yoga documentary *Enlighten Up!*, where a skeptical Jewish journalist tries to find inner peace on a voyage through the world of yoga. That hit way too close to home. Then you had the "Inappropriate Yoga Guy," whose hilarious YouTube videos had racked up a million hits. Will Ferrell's *SNL* sketch about achieving a yoga pose where he could suck his own dick had been making the rounds for almost a decade. They were doing yoga on *The Office*. Scarlett Johansson played a yoga teacher in *He's Just Not That into You*. *Couples Retreat* had that long scene with the loin-cloth clad Fabio lookalike yoga teacher. Scott Bakula was playing a yoga teacher on *Men of a Certain Age*. If you wanted to go even further back, Jenna Elfman did yoga humor in the mid-'90s on *Dharma and Greg*, for fuck's sake. But at some point, something would tip the scales, no one would be interested in buying yoga material anymore, and that would mean another path blocked by the cruel hand of fate.

No, I thought. *Not this time.* There may be a lot of competition in the small and unimportant world of yoga comedy, but Karuna Yoga is *mine*.

And then I did it. I tore his application in half, folded up the halves, and tore them again, and again, and again, until there was nothing left but little shreds. When this was done, I went outside to the Dumpster and put half the pieces in one side and half in another. I wadded a few of the pieces into a ball and placed them in my mouth, mashing them into an unrecognizable pulp with my saliva. I had to destroy all the evidence.

I went back inside and immediately felt horrible. My conscience began to scream. That had been one of the most quietly venal acts of my life.

I went home, put the kid to bed, and was doing the dishes when I called Regina into the kitchen.

"I did something bad," I said.

She sighed.

"What now?"

I told her.

"Do you really think you're not going to get found out?" she said.

"No," I said. "But . . ."

"Dude, the universe tested you, and you totally fucked it! You have to make this right."

"I can do that."

"Look, I understand the impulse. This is a competitive town. But that's no way to win."

"I know."

"Seriously, you could get into big trouble."

Envy, that most negative of emotions, had bubbled to the surface of my consciousness and caused me to do a wrong thing. It constantly threatened to upset the apple cart of my relative placidity. Those Morrissey lyrics, about hating our friends when they become successful, came to mind. The bigger the success, the greater threat posed by envy. As I wrote a few dozen pages ago, I've spent time publicly destroying other writers' books while in the grips of an alcohol-soaked, jealous rage. One of my favorite targets in that period was *Everything Is Illuminated* by Jonathan Safran Foer, who, immediately upon the book's publication, became the hot Jewish voice of his generation, a spot that I'd (unrealistically and without merit) been hoping to claim for myself.

If I'd been eighteen years old at an open mic, this behavior would have made some sense, but it was no activity for a reasonably accomplished man in his thirties. Also, not surprisingly, this occurred before I'd discovered yoga. Later, I read the *Yoga Sutras,* the philosophical basis for most modern yoga traditions. *Sutra* number 33, in the Desikachar translation, spells out the proper mental framework. In daily life, he says, we see people around who are happier than we are, and also people who are less happy. No matter our usual attitudes, we should be "pleased with others who are happier than ourselves, compassionate toward those who are unhappy," and "joyful with those doing praiseworthy things." This will leave our minds "very tranquil."

According to the *sutras,* the real obstacle to human happiness is *avidya,* or misperception, not seeing things the way they truly are. Of all the unproductive emotions in the world, none is worse for the soul, none more toxic to creative output, than envy. It will burn hot and fast for a short time, but when it flames out, it leaves a confused, miserable husk of a person in its wake. Do your own work, the *sutras* say, and don't let other people's work ripple your waters. Their business, whether you choose to enjoy it or not, has nothing to do with you.

So finally, after years of dedicated yoga practice, I'd begun to see, for instance, that while *Everything Is Illuminated* definitely isn't one of my favorite books, its creator could still be a well-meaning vegetarian force for good in the world. Any anger that I once had toward the book, and the author, mostly came from my misperception of it as a threat to my own imagined literary dominance.

And thus the impulse to destroy books began to leave my body, and my mind.

I try to remember this every time a friend of mine becomes successful, Morrissey notwithstanding. So when my former literary agent suddenly emerges as a regular character on *The Daily Show* and gets cast in one of the most successful TV ad campaigns of all time, I can feel happy for him, because he's a great guy who deserves all the odd success that comes his way. When a book that I blurb becomes a runaway global bestseller, I can send a hearty congratulatory email to the writer and invite him out for a drink, hoping that he'll pay. And when Dave Eggers, with whom I acted out a very public psychodrama in the first half of this decade, raises countless dollars for vital causes through writing books of extremely high quality, I can say, very quietly, "Good for him" instead of asking, "Why not me?" Then I can go back to my busy schedule of playing Civilization on my iPhone.

But on that night I tore up some kid's *seva* application, I'd only just begun to grapple with these searingly neurotic issues. After I talked to my wife, I began my attempts to writhe my way out of envy's alluring grip. I went downstairs. Fortunately, the guy was on Facebook. I wrote to him:

"Hey. It's Neal Pollack, the former *Reader* employee who was working the desk tonight at Karuna. I wanted to let you know that I misplaced your application. I have no idea where it went. There was a big rush for the 6:30 class, and I had to run a bunch of credit cards, and it vanished in the shuffle. I'm going to email the owner to tell her, but I think it's best that you come in and fill out another one . . . I'm really sorry for the hassle, man. I owe you a beer."

From there, I tried to deploy a more innocent deflection strategy. I said that Karuna is "a really nice studio with great teachers and cool, sincere students." Nothing topped it "in terms of high-quality yoga instruction and laid-back attitude." But as far as wacky characters went, I said, there were several other studios in the neighborhood that were better sources. I then named a bunch of studios that I'd never visited.

When that was done, I wrote to the studio owner:

"A guy stopped by the studio around 6 PM to turn in a SEVA application. Then I ended up doing some credit card transactions for Lauren's class. When the smoke cleared, I'd completely misplaced his application. I searched high and low but couldn't find it anywhere. So it's probably in the studio somewhere, but I have no idea where. . . . I already contacted him on Facebook (it was definitely him), so he knows to come in and request another application if he's still interested. I'm really sorry about this . . . I don't know where my head was tonight. I imagine you'll be hearing from him soon. Thanks for your patience. I'm sure you've dealt with worse."

The next day, the guy wrote me back:

"Thanks for the heads up. I will drop by and fill out another app. And thanks for the tips on the other, more 'eccentric,' studios around town. Great meeting you."

He included a friend request.

A few weeks later, he started working a regular shift on Saturdays at Karuna. But by then, my mind had righted itself. For help, I'd sought guidance from a handy paperback called *1001 Pearls of Yoga Wisdom*. How would the masters deal with such a situation, I wondered. I found this one from the great Swami Sivananda: "There is no end of craving. Hence contentment alone is the best way to happiness. Therefore, acquire contentment."

Yes, envy was bad, particularly combined with covetousness. That guy could write a dozen yoga pilots for all I cared. If one hit, I'd even think about being happy for him. I had everything I wanted and needed, right now.

A couple of days later, I heard back from Karuna's owner:

"Thanks for the update," she wrote. "No worries. I am glad that you are here at the studio taking care of the community."

8

Have Mat, Will Travel

In the yoga tradition, nothing is more important than the student-teacher relationship. Each student is supposed to have one teacher. They form a sacred bond through hard work, philosophical conversation, and disciplined study. The great Krishnamacharya, the man most indirectly responsible for the ongoing yoga boom in the West, spent nearly a decade in a Tibetan cave learning from a *sadhu*, or holy man. And this was *after* he'd obtained the equivalent of several PhDs in Vedic language and literature.

But this wasn't India, or Tibet, and I had no discipline. I

lived in the yoga equivalent of Temptation Island. Los Angeles had so many teachers who had so much to teach. A wise man with whom I later studied the *sutras* had this to say about my many yoga options: "You can go to McDonald's, and, yes, technically it's food. You can definitely eat there and feel full when you're done. But is it really good for you?" In other words, seeking advice from many of these teachers wasn't going to help. If it walked like yoga and quacked like yoga, it wasn't necessarily yoga.

I didn't totally agree with him. There are some teachers who specialize in certain aspects of the yoga tradition, and who do them better than others. Some days, you just want a good aerobic workout. Other times, you're just looking to relax. Perhaps you want to learn breathing or meditation techniques. Occasionally a friend is teaching a class and you want to support them so they (and you) don't feel lonely. The yoga mall is here, so why not go shopping?

But malls quickly become alienating and annoying. If you stay in them too long, they begin to drive you crazy. At some point, an endless search for the next big yoga thing just becomes another manifestation of the unfocused mind. It certainly happened to me; shiny yoga objects kept blinking, distracting me from the true nature of reality. McDonald's was everywhere, I kept eating, and I was starving.

One afternoon, as I picked my son up from school, he handed me a piece of art he'd made. It involved the usual subject matter: space robots fighting one another over candy. The boy was about to turn six, so this is what occupied his mind.

The drawing was so enthralling that I didn't see the stone bench in front of me. I stumbled, catching myself with my left hand. This kept my head from smacking into the bench, but the art blew away in the autumn breeze.

I felt a sharp pain at the base of my left ring finger. It had been bothering me all week during yoga practice, and now I began to worry that I'd broken a bone, pulled a muscle, or snapped some part of my body that I previously hadn't known existed.

My finger was still throbbing when I got home. I put it on ice. With my good hand, I pecked out an email to Mara, telling her about my injury and saying that I was going to "bow out" for the time being. She wrote back:

"My opinion is that it is always better to do the practice, even with injuries. It teaches us to be even more mindful and kind toward this lovely, imperfect form of ours.

"I've been practicing through a shoulder injury for about a year now, and it is really interesting the stuff that it brings up. Like the temper tantrum that my ego throws when I can't do all my *chatarangas*, for instance. But what's amazing is that my practice is still growing—even though I feel like a freakin' cripple some days! STILL I'm getting stronger and more refined in my *asanas*. So, your choice of course. But I say come and just be prepared to communicate slowly and clearly with the part of yourself that wants to do too much."

Curse Mara and her yogic wisdom! I forwarded the email to Regina, who took exception.

"Dude," she wrote me back. "Don't be stupid. Your HAND is FUCKED up. Take a one-day break. For chrissakes."

I went upstairs so we could have this argument in person.

"Nah," I said. "I think I'm going to practice tomorrow."

"You're going to listen to your yoga teacher instead of your wife."

"Uh-huh."

"I don't like that."

"Not my problem."

"You either do yoga or go to the doctor," she said. "You can't do both."

"I'm gonna do whatever the hell I want," I said.

"I'm sure you will."

I decided I would go to yoga, but I wanted to stay married, so I took the weekend off from practicing and I made a doctor's appointment for the following Monday. They took X-rays and determined that I had a sprained finger tendon. That's the kind of injury that keeps a guy out of the lineup for a couple of days, not weeks or months, and they treated it accordingly. He ran a "cold laser" over the damaged area for a while, though it might have been a museum pointer for all I knew. Regardless, it didn't hurt worse. The doctor told me to yank on the affected knuckle as often as possible. This, he said, would lubricate the joint and speed up the healing process. Then he gave me a chiropractic adjustment and let me lay on a motorized massage table for a while.

By the following week, I was totally better, and Mara showed me how to do something. I sat cross-legged and leaned forward with my elbows bent. I unfolded my legs smoothly and thrust them out behind me. Then I lowered myself, elbows still bent, and swooped upward into upward-facing dog. This was the great *chataranga dhandasana*, the core move of all *hatha* yoga. I'd finally learned how to execute it semi-properly.

When I finished, I sat on my mat for a while, feeling proud of myself.

"What asana is this?" Mara asked. "Lazy asana? Sit on your butt asana? Pick your toes asana?"

I looked down and realized that I actually *had* been picking lint out of my toes.

"Give me a break, woman," I said. "I just jumped back out of seated!"

She laughed and moved on to torturing her next victim. In fact, unbeknownst to me, but knownst to her, I was just taking a shortcut to moving back into *chataranga* from seated position, and I was nowhere near the actual pose. Over the next year, I spent a lot of time straining and grunting with my hands on blocks, trying to lift my butt off the floor so I could excute the move properly, and I achieved very limited results. No wonder Mara had laughed.

I might practice yoga for three lifetimes and probably not find another teacher who'd allow me to talk to her like that. But I couldn't spend my entire life in Mara's little underground yoga nest, could I? There was a big wide yoga world, and I'd barely seen anything. I thought I could do *chataranga* now. Soon, I might even be able to do *chataranga* out of crow pose. A desire ran strong in me: I wanted to sling my earth-toned yoga mat bag over my shoulder and head on down the road. It was time to share my emerging best self with the rest of humanity.

One day, I told Mara that I needed to move along. She seemed to understand.

"Stop by once in a while," she said. "I'll give you special dispensation."

"Thank you," I said. "I'm a little nervous."

"You're definitely ready," she said, with the confident tone of someone who knew I'd be back.

I could snatch the pebble from her hand.

Time for me to leave.

For the next few months, I wandered the yogascape like a clueless British tourist in Amsterdam's red-light district: I entered rooms that I had no business being in, and I almost always had a disappointing headache when I was done.

It started close to home. Several studios in my neighborhood offered special deals, like ten days of consecutive yoga for only twenty bucks. At one studio, I continually drew the same substitute teacher, a pregnant woman who referred to herself as a "passionate social worker." She had us practice many positions on our fingertips, which hurt like hell and made me angry. I did take one Sunday class with a kind, lanky dude named Billy. He gave me good tips on my *trikanasana*. But it wasn't enough for me to run the credit card there again.

At another studio, I practiced with a sexy young hipster whose teaching goals appeared to be playing the coolest mix of music imaginable and having her students do many impossible push-up variations. One day before class started, she asked us to name our "album of the year." I said The Arcade Fire's latest, not because I'd actually heard the album, but because I'd seen it mentioned on various websites. In any case, I wondered, what did my album of the year have to do with yoga? Patty never asked us what music we liked. She just played the same songs every week whether we liked them or not.

Against my better judgment, I also took classes in Phoenix. I'd been visiting my parents there a lot more often since I'd moved to L.A. Where I'd once resented Phoenix because it always has been and always will be a soulless sinkhole of mediocrity, I now appreciated having pretty much unlimited access to a large, comfortable house with a pool in a quiet neighborhood surrounded by starkly beautiful Saguaro-dotted mountains. I began to understand the appeal of retirement. Also, there's nothing quite like having enthusiastic, free babysitters.

A ten-minute drive away from my parents' house was a studio. On my next visit I went there for a class. It had bleached-white walls and a boutique area bigger than my backyard. Middle-aged women walked around, wearing clothes made of money. Compared with this place, I practiced yoga in a not-up-to-code attic. I approached the desk.

"I'd like to take a class," I said.

"Have you been here before?" asked the desk lady.

"I have not."

"That'll be twenty dollars."

"TWENTY DOLLARS?" I said. "Are you fucking joking?"

"Nope."

"That's too expensive."

"You could buy an OmPass," she said.

"What's an OmPass?"

An OmPass is sort of like a yoga frequent-filer miles program where you get free-class coupons at local participating studios, and 20 to 30 percent "traveler discounts" at studios in other cities. The OmPass website also offers gift cards, personal stories from "Celebrity OmStars" that seem to be a low-rent form of yoga payola, a Q&A section with OmPass' resident yoga expert "Posemaster K," a video of Russell Simmons doing various poses while spouting philosophy, and a "business opportunity" for studios to affiliate themselves with OmPass for the low, low activation price of $99, which includes a Free Organic OmPass Wood Display Stand. Perhaps this was what Mara meant by capitalist yoga.

I paid $19.95 for my OmPass, which reduced my class price to something in the somewhat more reasonable sixteen-dollar range. Then I went to the class. For the next hour and a half, a short man with a smug grin led me, along with about forty hard-core yoga monkeys in skin-tight outfits, through a tough Power Yoga workout that included a pose that he annoyingly called "Wild Thing." *What was next*, I thought, *"Brown Sugar?" How about "Aqualung?" Or "Mr. Roboto?"* That would be a cool name for a pose, too.

Then it came time for *savasana*. "You know what to do," the teacher said. I closed my eyes and attempted to rest. All around me, I heard the rustling of mats. Maybe three minutes passed until I came out of my corpse. I looked around. One other person was still lying down. Other than that, the room was empty except for a guy giving a woman a massage. The teacher couldn't be found. I actually felt insulted. You're supposed to *hold down* the room during *savasana*, not walk out on your students. What a load, though it wasn't as bad as the next time I took a class at that studio, where the teacher had us go into deep relaxation accompanied by a live recording of Jimmy Cliff singing *Many Rivers to Cross.*

As I went on book tours or the occasional freelance magazine assignment, I started bringing my yoga mat with me. It became a mandatory part of every trip; before I left, I did an extended online search for classes near where I was staying, and tried to shape my schedule around the classes I wanted to take. I'd been traveling for decades and had never thought about yoga. Now, suddenly, yoga seemed to be everywhere, and I could sense its presence. I'd developed yogadar.

My studies took me to a third-floor walkup in the middle of a Chicago light-industrial zone, and the deck of the Standard Hotel in Miami Beach. I took a class in Toronto when it was fifteen below outside, and several while attending my cousin's wedding on Nantucket. Some of the classes were better than others, but it was always nice to have something familiar in a strange setting that was also something strange in a familiar setting.

For one overnight trip to San Francisco, I stuffed clean underwear, a T-shirt, a pair of socks, a toothbrush, toothpaste, and deodorant into my mat bag, and announced to Regina that I wasn't taking a suitcase.

"Wow," she said. "You are just so amazing."

Mock me all you want, wife, I thought. *Your snide critiques mean nothing to me. I'm a bona fide yoga gypsy.*

When I got to San Francisco, the only class I could fit into my schedule was something around lunchtime at a local studio chain. The teacher was a "substitute," which is generally yoga-teacher code for "someone not experienced enough yet to have their own class." She was very cute and perky, though.

"The first thing you should know about me," she said, "is that I'm a renegade yogi."

Uh-oh.

"*Renegade*, like Lorenzo Lamas?" I said to the woman on the mat next to me. "Where's her motorcycle?"

The woman didn't respond.

The teacher devoted much of the class to showing us a yoga move that she'd made up *all by herself*. She called it the "swoosh swoosh," and you can just imagine. Instead, I stayed in warrior two for a few seconds longer.

Later in class she came up to me and said, "Nice forearm stand, dude!" I felt bad for having thought mean things about her. But I still wasn't going to do the swoosh swoosh.

One Monday afternoon, after a vigorous morning practice, I hopped a JetBlue flight from Burbank to JFK. About halfway through, while coming back from the privy at the front of the plane, I noticed a familiar green-and-gold box of Guyaki sitting on the galley shelf.

"Excuse me," I said to the flight attendant. "Is that *yerba mate*?"

"It certainly is," she said, in an accent that could only have come from the South. "Would you like some?"

"Oh, yes," I said.

"I like it so much better than coffee," she said. "Coffee makes me crazy."

"Me, too," I said. "*Mate* is a nice, smooth high."

"Definitely," she said. "Do you want some soy milk with it?"

My yogadar was tingling.

The *mate* went through my system quickly, and I was back at the can before too long. When I came out, I noticed that the flight attendant had two issues of *Yoga Journal* open on her lap. She was going through them with a highlighter, and was also taking notes.

"Huh," I said. "You're reading *Yoga Journal*."

"Yeah," she said. "It's like getting a free yoga class."

"You practice?"

"Actually, I teach. I'm taking notes for a monthly column I write for my studio's newsletter."

Do tell.

She'd done a two-hundred-hour certification with Baron Baptiste, the internationally renowned creator of "Power Vinyasa Yoga" and the author of *My Daddy Is a Pretzel*. She now taught regularly at her neighborhood studio in Charlotte. She did *hatha* classes, but her special calling, she said, was prenatal yoga. She'd done that when she was pregnant, and it had changed her life. Now, she said, her eighteen-month-old daughter was her "greatest teacher" and a "natural yogi."

Normally, I'm pretty skeptical when people say they learn from their children. The only thing I'd learned from my son was how to blackmail someone into taking a shower. But in the spirit of yogic goodness, I nodded and smiled.

"It must be really hard keeping a yoga mindset on an airplane," I said.

"Oh, you have no idea," she said. "When I see people getting upset over little things that don't matter, I want to tell them to detach. It would really help them. But I'd probably get fired if I did that."

Well, that sounded juicy. Maybe she had one of those apocryphal stories of an angry businessman getting drunk and throwing his own feces into economy class. I fished for gossip.

"Anything specific you want to talk about?"

"I'd prefer not."

"Lord knows I have trouble detaching when *I'm* flying," I said, throwing out another line.

"So do I," she said. "Every moment is a struggle."

"It's hard to see the world with fresh eyes," I added. "There are so many distractions."

"It's so true," she said. "If only everyone could see that."

"I didn't," I said. "Before yoga."

We continued like this for quite a while, not talking about anything concrete, mostly just quoting randomly from the *sutras* and rhapsodizing about yoga's magic transformational power. She knew more than I did, but I didn't embarrass myself. Suddenly, I realized that I was sitting cross-legged at the front of an airplane, having a fairly sincere metaphysical discussion with a flight attendant. Though we'd never practiced together and never would, at that moment it felt like yoga had sealed us together with a powerful, almost unbreakable bond.

"Would you listen to us?" I said. "We sound like a couple of fundamentalist Christians talking about how we've seen the light."

"You're right," she said. "It really makes the time pass, doesn't it?"

"Time is but an abstraction when you can gaze into eternity," I said.

"Indeed," she said.

The captain turned on the fasten seat belt sign.

A few minutes later, as I dragged my carry-on down the aisle, I turned to my new friend, put my hands together in prayer position at my heart center, and bowed, monk-like.

"Namaste," I said to her.

She bowed back.

"Namaste," she said.

"So is this your usual route?" I asked.

"Nah," she said. "But we'll see each other again."

That was doubtful, but I didn't care.

I turned away, pulled my mothballed pea coat collar up across my ugly sweater, adjusted my Russian-style hat that had been fashionable ten years earlier when I'd last lived in a cold climate, and stepped off the plane. My heart felt full. That was how I'd once connected with people all the time, when I was young and free, before time and the world made me bitter and hairy and flatulent. There had been no artifice on that plane, no judgment, just pure joy and good wishes. I'd made a profound human connection at thirty-five thousand feet, seen into the essence of another human soul. Could my best self have returned at last?

If so, New York would test it mightily.

New York City is a hard place for someone not from New York City to do yoga. As with everything else, New Yorkers are so much more serious and intense about yoga than ordinary people, and they do it so much better. At one point early in my fascinating voyage of self-discovery, I ran into a New York friend at a yoga class in L.A. She said, "Oh, I didn't know you were doing yoga! Do you do it once or twice a day?" If by "day" she meant "week," then the answer was once.

Even though they continue to practice with the obsession of borderline mental patients chewing their cuticles, most New Yorkers have considered yoga to be over since the exact date that they wrote a magazine article or blogpost on the subject. It's the only place on Earth that supports a serious yoga backlash, represented by the popular FUCK YOGA T-shirts that you see on *Sex and the City* reruns. New York performer Mike Albo sums up their attitude perfectly: "Everybody's doing yoga now," he says. "Fat people, old people . . . retarded people." In other words, have your little yoga experience if you must, but if your practice doesn't predate Madonna's, or at least Russell Simmons', then it doesn't really count.

Yoga inspires flaky goofball capitalism everywhere, but nowhere on Earth is the madness as complete in New York. In a *New York Magazine* article, Vanessa Grigoriadis had this to say about the scene in 2001: "Once the domain of hippies and Californians, yoga has become a New York obsession over the past few years . . . the goal may be egolessness, but that hasn't stopped entrepreneurs from creating, branding, and trademarking their very own types of yoga. It's a crowded market, so each studio has to have a gimmick: There are yoga centers for young seekers, for the physically insatiable, for those who want to avoid a scene. There's even a Buddhist yoga studio, Om, run by Cyndi Lee, a former choreographer who crafted the moves for Cyndi Lauper's 'Girls Just Want to Have Fun' video."

One Thursday evening in Manhattan, I went to a class taught by an almost impossibly sexy woman in her early forties. Most of the other students were *also* sexy women in their thirties and forties. Sometimes, when you're in New York, it's hard to imagine that the city is home to any other type of person. Many of the students brought roses for their teacher and laid them on her harmonium. "OH, THANK YOU!" she exclaimed, when she made her big entrance at 6:30 PM, on the nose. "They smell so nice!"

Devotional guru offerings were anathema to the way I operated. I mean, Patty's students loved her and all, but the closest they ever came to worship was buying her a cup of coffee after class. The only offering I'd ever seen Mara receive was a packet of Pop Rocks, which she placed in an incense burner and didn't touch for months. I wondered if this teacher would have been so friendly if her students *hadn't* brought her flowers.

She sat down cross-legged at her harmonium and began the evening's talk.

"In our lineage," she said, "there's a concept that we know of as *samskara*. Now, many of you know what that means, right. What does it mean?"

About three-quarters of the room said, in unison, "misery!"

"That's right. Misery. Mundane existence. And we have to deal with that, right? Every day. So we spend a lot of time trying to make ourselves happy. If you're anything like me, from the moment you wake up in the morning until the moment you go to bed, all you think about is how to make yourself happy. What can I wear? What can I eat? What can I watch on TV?"

Jesus Christ, lady, I thought. *Can we just do some poses already?* But it wasn't time for that yet.

"You try to make yourself happy," she continued. "But our teachers say that the amount of your happiness is totally dependent on the amount of happiness you give other people. Still, we try to seek *refuge* in our own happiness. It's an important concept, refuge. It's a cloak from the true self."

She asked the gathered: "What things do you seek refuge in that you think will make you happy?"

The answers came readily:

"Shopping!"

"Clothes!"

"Alcohol!"

"Heroin!"

"Heroin?" said the teacher.

"Only on the weekends," said the student.

The entire class laughed, not in a "that's so absurd" way, but in a "that's so familiar" way.

"You know that won't make you happy," the teacher said. "Relationships won't make you happy either. And marriage? Forget about it. We all know that marriage doesn't get you away from life's problems. If anything, it creates *more* problems. Has anyone in here been married more than once?"

No hands went up. *Whoa,* I thought. *What's the backstory behind that question?*

"Has anyone here been married *once*?"

Mine was one of about a half-dozen raised hands. We hadn't even started the *asana* yet, and I already felt tired.

On another afternoon in New York, I found myself on a street corner in midtown, licking salt off a slightly burned soft pretzel. I gazed about in a wondering daze, transfixed by the LCD nightmare. Time seemed to stop for me just then, as though I were Dr. Manhattan from *Watchmen*, only without the continually erect blue penis. Suddenly, I knew that everything in Times Square—the breeze-blown fliers for some outlier porn shop, the vaguely contraband luggage stores, the endlessly replicated advertisments for TV shows that never had a prayer, even the tourists from Nebraska—was part of a larger cosmic reality whose boundaries we can't begin to perceive. The power of the universe, I realized, is transcendent, infinite, all-knowing, beautiful beyond measure. I quaked at the awesome kindness of its eternal might.

This, in yoga terms, is called *Samadhi*, the divine perception of universal consciousness, though the realization may have come to me because I was in the middle of a five-day drug bender. I'd bought some full-melt *sativa* hash capsules at my neighborhood medical-marijuana dispensary before coming to town, had taken two caps before getting on the plane, and had refried my brain first thing three consecutive mornings. Visions like these were happening regularly now; my synapses had begun to fray around the edges.

While there's no specific verse in the *Yoga Sutras* about overindulging one's desire for hash, it does teach moderation in all things and tells you not to become too attached to objects of pleasure. Such attachments just lead to more suffering. All I needed was to lie down for a couple of hours with a wet washcloth over my face, but I'd made plans to meet a friend for an early evening yoga class at her favorite studio. She was excited to share this experience with me. Doing yoga at this place, she said, had made her life so much better.

"Fuck yeah!" I said, when she asked me. "I love yoga!"

Jivamukti was her studio of choice. Those of you who know about yoga just gave a little moan, or gasp, or cheer of recognition, but for those of you who don't, Jivamukti (a Sanskrit word that means "liberation while living") is a yoga method that combines physical postures with scriptural study, music, chanting, meditation, animal rights, veganism, environmentalism, and political activism. David Life and Sharon Gannon, the method's founders, were obscure downtown Manhattan avant-garde theater performers before they began their new careers teaching yoga to recovering junkies in a tiny room in the East Village. They opened their first Jivamukti studio in 1990. Soon after, Life took a vow of poverty, celibacy, and simplicity and changed his name to Swami Bodhananda. This lasted until 1993. "It just didn't work in New York," he said in a magazine profile. "People were treating me like a guru, and I never wanted to be that."

But he achieved a kind of guru-hood nonetheless, and his fame has spread throughout the world. There are now two Jivamukti centers in New York, and one each in Toronto, Munich, London, and Charleston, South Carolina. The Jivamukti website features devotional quotes from Christy Turlington and Sting. According to the *New York Times*, "Without Jivamukti, yoga in the United States would still be the obscure practice of a few devotees."

Yoga at Jivamukti is very serious and requires a deeper commitment than, say, taking a class once a week at the local YMCA. The Jivamukti website says, "We promote the

educational aspect of the practice and give students access
to where these ideas have come from. Each class focuses on
a theme, which is supported by Sanskrit chanting, readings,
references to scriptural texts, music (from the Beatles to
Moby), spoken word, asana sequencing and yogic breathing
practices. The average Jivamukti student is more educated
about the philosophy of yoga than most yoga teachers."

The practice is adored by many, is considered the height
of pretension on Earth by others, and owns a special place
in the New York yoga backlash. Later, when I mentioned
it to a friend, she referred to it as "Jive-Ass Monkey." Of
course, I knew none of this when I got off the elevator and
entered the Jivamukti den, high as an Underdog balloon. I
was planning to simply take another class on another chilly
spring afternoon. My friend and I would do some yoga,
towel off in separate locker rooms, and then go get some
tasty noodle soup.

I entered a room the size of a soccer pitch. Students set
up their mats so they were nearly touching, in rows of ten.
My preference would have been to hide in the middle-back.
That way, the teacher might forget about me. But my friend
plopped down in the front row, close to the door, so I had
to splay next to her. Across the aisle from us, an equally
deep number of full rows took shape, like an opposing pha-
lanx in some sort of yoga war. I was used to studying in
small rooms with no more than twenty people, and often
fewer than ten. This felt about as intimate as getting on the
subway.

Several short women wearing white, v-neck blouses
walked around the room, hands behind their backs, examining the scene. They looked kind of like massage therapists

to me. I grew hopeful—a massage sounded pretty good. *Maybe I shouldn't do yoga today,* I thought. *Maybe I should get a massage instead.*

The instructor entered. She was tall and lithe, and she moved with a healthy, almost ethereal confidence. A few freckles, perfectly placed, dotted her angular face. You've had many yoga instructors who've looked like her, except that she was hotter by a degree of ten. She walked into the center of the room.

"OK, the thing you have to understand about the world," she said, "is that most people are totally selfish, right?"

Well, that was always a good conversation starter.

"If you're being selfish," she continued, "if you're only thinking about yourself, then you're hurting the world. And what you have to understand, you guys, is that the *choices* you make, right, totally affect the *environment*. And that you have a responsibility to the world to make the right choices."

Usually, my yoga teachers never gave a rap longer than, "I've had kind of a rough day, and I've been thinking I need some yoga to center myself, so let's get started." But this went on and on. I wasn't then aware that Jivamukti instructors are required to give a fifteen-minute *dharma* lecture before class. They're told to stress the *yamas,* or codes of conduct, for yogic living. These include: Non-harming, non-stealing, non-lying, non-attachment, and the always-unpopular celibacy. The studio's politics are never far away, either. Sharon Gannon, after all, once published a book called *Cats and Dogs Are People Too.*

"I like to think of myself as an ethical vegan," the teacher continued. "And that informs my yoga practice, and it helps me to heal the world. Did you know, you guys, that research has shown if you eat meat, you're doing more harm to the environment than if you drive an SUV? Think about that while you're doing your yoga. If 98 percent of the people who drove SUVs stopped driving them tomorrow, it still wouldn't help the environment because of all the damage that meat-eaters do. So when you're eating meat, think about all the harm you're doing to the world because you're selfish and greedy and don't think about others."

This particular *dharma* lecture confused me. Weren't yoga teachers supposed to present themselves as humble servants of a higher power rather than moral paragons above reproach or laughter? Also, while I've had some raw-food episodes in my life, and understand and appreciate the philosophy behind veganism, her science was almost as faulty as her manner was condescending. Someone needed to take her down a notch. The right time to do it, I figured, was during a yoga class attended by a hundred of her followers, while I was toasted to the nines.

"Bullshit!" I said.

My friend looked at me, pained and nervous, pleading with her eyes for me to stop. The teacher heard because she was right in front of me.

"If someone disagrees with what I'm saying," she said, "they're obviously not well-informed and are speaking from a position of insecurity."

"I'm not the *only* one," I mumbled under my breath.

This wasn't going to go well.

She huffed haughtily and resumed her *dharma* talk.

Finally, our physical practice began. It pushed way

beyond any level I could handle. The flow moved too fast, and many of the positions were new to me. I stumbled around, flinging sweat off my head onto other people's mats, huffing and sighing. The instructor, by now, had me in her crosshairs. She kept giving me adjustments, though the most effective adjustment might have been to put me in a chair and leave me there.

"Maybe you should practice a little bit before you start criticizing," she said.

"Maybe I should."

"Maybe you should."

"That's what I just said."

She walked away. I don't think I was her type of student. Then again, I'd yet to find a yoga teacher who was naturally drawn to sarcastic, incompetent fat-asses. I closed my eyes and tried to focus on the practice. Then the teacher's voice lowered about two octaves, and she started talking much more slowly. In fact, it sounded like another voice altogether.

"Now," said the voice, "keep your heart open—wide open—and move your shoulder blades apart as you slide your hands into warrior two."

I opened my eyes as I moved into the pose. One of the women in white was now guiding the practice. This teacher had *assistants*, for god's sake.

"Is this some sort of fucking cult?" I said.

My friend, realizing she'd made a horrible mistake by inviting me, drew her lips together with a loud SHHHH.

Yoga teachers don't need assistants, I thought. Sure, if you're Patthabi Jois or B. K. S. Iyengar or some other nonagenarian whose near-divine presence has made prac-

tice possible for millions of people, you've earned the right
to sit quietly while your senior disciples do the heavy lifting. But for the love of Krishna, if you're a sexy Manhattan
broad at the height of your powers, don't pawn your extra
vinyasas off on underlings!

At some point, after she'd retaken control of the tiller,
the instructor made a joke. By now, we were doing the
seated poses, so I could at least breathe. I don't remember
the joke, but, for some reason, I laughed.

"Oh, so the *comedian* thinks I'm funny," she said. "I
must be doing something right."

Lady, I'm no comedian, I thought. *I'm a comic writer.*
There's a difference.

Finally, we got to *savasana*. Boy, did I need it. I lay
down on my rental mat and prepared for ten minutes or
so of sweet relief from the nightmarish yoga journey I'd
just endured. Then I heard a voice. Some sort of recording
was being played. The voice was British, with the hint of a
Middle Eastern accent, and as preachy as Noam Chomsky
being interviewed by a college-newspaper editor.

"The United Nations estimates," said the voice, "that
more than four hundred thousand people have died in Iraq
since the start of the Gulf War. The estimated profits made
by U.S. corporations since that time have equaled . . ."

"*Are you fucking kidding me?*" I said.

"Please don't do this," said my friend, rapidly becoming
my former friend.

"In 1980," said the tape, "Saddam Hussein met with
Donald Rumsfeld . . ."

I stormed out, mat in hand. Sure, I was against the war
in Iraq and all, really against it, big time. I'd organized a

group to march against George W. Bush's first inauguration, for god's sake. My lefty bonafides didn't need proving.
But the last thing I needed to hear during *savasana* was a
recitation of recent U.S. war crimes in the Middle East.

I went into the lobby and gave the desk clerk the crazy
druggie eye.

"WHO THE FUCK DOES THAT TEACHER THINK
SHE IS?" I said.

The desk people ignored me.

"I WANT TO FILE A COMPLAINT!"

Still, they ignored me.

"THAT WAS AWFUL, WHAT WENT ON IN THERE!
ALL THE POLITICAL RANTING! THIS IS YOGA, GOD-
DAMMIT! I CAN'T BELIEVE IT! THIS PLACE IS A
FUCKING NIGHTMARE!"

It didn't occur to me that the people working behind
the desk at Jivamukti might side with the teacher in any dis-
agreement. But I'm not one to keep my displeasure bottled.

"FUCK!" I shouted.

I turned to the woman behind the desk.

"Do you need me to clean my yoga mat?" I said. "It's
very sweaty."

"We'll take care of it," she said.

Five minutes later, my now former friend came out of
class. We went downstairs to the street.

"I can't believe you did that," she said.

"That fucking bitch," I said.

"I don't care if you disagreed with her. This place is important to me, and you embarrassed me in class."

"But . . ."

"That was totally humiliating for me."

My friend wanted an apology. So, about six months later, I emailed her one. The incident continued to trouble me, though. The teacher had preached, didactically and unpleasantly. But what I'd done in response, I finally realized, had been totally wrong and disrespectful. I'd been so caught up in my own anger and cynical judgment that I'd forgotten to draw any knowledge at all from my experience. It took months for me to look Jivamukti up online, to understand what I'd been facing. I'd gone blindly into one of the founding studios of modern yoga, thrown a fit worthy of a toddler so far gone that no shiny object could distract him from his rage, and left with nothing in return.

Before the yoga, I'd behaved that way fairly often. It was about as far from my best self as I could get. In fact, I'd even go so far as to call it my *bad self.* But even serious yogis, I was learning, are often tempted to get down with their bad selves. I now realized that couldn't ever stop my bad self from manifesting, not entirely. Trying to contain it was the true yoga practice, the real discipline and dedication, and maybe if I went back to my regular teachers, instead of wandering hither and yon looking for something that I didn't even need, they could help me. But I still had many more thousands of miles to travel. The distracting objects were about to get much shinier.

9

On the Cover of *Yoga Journal*

The first recorded incidence of yoga in the United States occurred at the 1893 Parliament of World Religions in Chicago. On the not-yet-apocryphal date of September 11, the honored Indian guest Swami Vivekananda addressed the gathering as "Sisters and Brothers of America." According to published reports, the crowd, upon hearing these five words, was so moved by the depth of Vivekananda's sincerity that it gave him a rapturous three-minute standing ovation. When that died down, the Swami responded, "It fills my heart with joy unspeakable to rise in response to the warm and cordial welcome which you have given us . . ."

Yoga in America was off to a good start.

The Swami's speech was short but profound: "Sectarianism, bigotry, and its horrible descendant, fanaticism, have long possessed this beautiful Earth. They have filled the earth with violence, drenched it often and often with human blood, destroyed civilization, and sent whole nations to despair. Had it not been for these horrible demons, human society would be far more advanced than it is now ... But their time is come; and I fervently hope that the bell that tolled this morning in honor of this convention may be the death-knell of all fanaticism, of all persecutions with the sword or with the pen, and of all uncharitable feelings between persons wending their way to the same goal."

This prediction proved a bit off the mark. Regardless, yoga continued along its quiet path in the West. In 1920 Paramahansa Yogananda came to Boston, founded the Self-Realization Fellowship, and later published *Autobiography of a Yogi*, still read today by college sophomores and aspiring yoga teachers everywhere. Any number of fakirs and charlatans found success in his wake, but then came *hatha*.

Physical yoga established its first true American beachhead in 1947, when Indra Devi, "the first lady of yoga" and beloved pupil of Sri Krishnamacharya, opened a studio in Hollywood, claiming as her students such stars as Gloria Swanson, Jennifer Jones, and Robert Ryan. No known photos exist of Jennifer Jones (who died in 2009) doing yoga in her prime, but if they did, I'd definitely be looking at them on the Internet right now.

The 1950s brought us Selvarajan Yesudian, whose book *Sport and Yoga* sold more than five hundred thousand copies and paved the way for dozens of annoying local-sports-section feature stories about football players doing yoga during training camp. In 1961, Richard Hittelman, who'd learned yoga from a Hindu janitor at a Catskills resort called Utopia, reached a larger audience than any yogi in history when he began hosting *Yoga for Health* on KQED-TV in Los Angeles. His books sold eight million copies and he traveled the world, teaching yoga poses in places like the old tennis courts in Grand Central Station. After that, he got divorced, founded a weird church, and died alone of cancer, saddling his ex-wife with a million-dollar IRS tax lien, thus proving that yoga guru-hood doesn't guarantee one a graceful third act.

Then came the late '60s, a time during which the American mind was tuned in to some pretty freaky channels. These were the glory days of the Maharishi Mahesh Yogi and his Transcendental Meditation, which inspired mar.y bad songs but also a few good ones, like "Across the Universe." Waves of joy were drifting through our open minds once Yogi Bhajan arrived in California with his *kundalini* yoga. Meanwhile, Swami Sivananda, from his high Himalayan perch, sent his disciples throughout the west. One of them, Swami Chidananda, got a hold of mild-mannered Lilias Folan and apparently instructed her to star on a popular PBS program throughout the 1970s. *Lilias, Yoga and You,* with its sexless unitards and monochromatic backgrounds, came to define physical yoga for a generation of well-meaning, Volvo-driving Woody Allen fans. Today, Lilias continues to teach yoga, mostly to senior citizens in Cincinnati.

Meanwhile, the seeds for yoga's true explosion in the West were sprouting back in India. Indra Devi may have come first, but two of Krishnamacharya's other star pupils had been building their own reputations for decades. In 1948, Sri K. Patthabi Jois opened his Ashtanga Yoga Research Institute in Mysore. A Belgian named Andre Van Lysebeth studied with him in the mid-1960s, and published a book called *Yoga, Self-Taught*. As that book caught on, Westerners began to travel to Mysore to study with the master, and gradually began bringing his teachings back to the states. Patthabi Jois made his first appearance on U.S. soil in the mid-'70s, at a studio in Encinitas, California.

Over in the city of Pune, Krishnamacharya's brother-in-law, B. K. S. Iyengar, had been perfecting his *own* soon-to-be famous method. In 1952, he met and befriended the violinist Yehudi Menuhin, who arranged for Iyengar to travel around Europe teaching yoga, bringing the practice to another swath of the West. When, in 1966, Iyengar published his bestselling classic *Light on Yoga*, all the ingredients were in place.

No one can exactly trace the moment that yoga became an unstoppable cultural force in the world of rich exercise addicts. Despite surges in popularity and great enthusiasm in certain pockets, it remained largely hidden from public view in the United States, practiced in smelly walkups and the backs of health-food stores from the East River to the Pacific. But before anyone could invent a machine to go back in time and stop them, Madonna and Gwyneth started doing Ashtanga and we were all fucked.

One minute, everyone trendy was Jazzercizing, and then, suddenly, yoga had become the ubiquitous $5.6 billion a year global industry that we simultaneously adore and loathe today. A *Sex and the City* episode featured the

"Yogasm." Iyengar and Jois had their portraits in *Vanity Fair.* In 1998, Chip Wilson, a passionate surfer and snowboarder, opened the first Lululemon Athletica retail store in the Kitsilano area of central Vancouver, finally realizing Swami Vivekananda's 105-year-old dream.

At some point very late in this history, I started writing for *Yoga Journal.*

Raymond Chandler once wrote that someone could live an entire life in Los Angeles and never get to the part where they make the movies. Sometimes it seemed like I was going to live one of those lives. My Hollywood dream—the one in which I made hundreds of millions of dollars by creating a TV show as lauded by critics as *Curb Your Enthusiasm,* but about parenting—had been deferred, by the WGA strike and by many other things too boring to elucidate, including my own incompetence.

Money was tight. I was ready to take any assignment, from anywhere. As an hour of great need approached, my friend, the last working magazine journalist on earth, got in touch. She'd received an email from an editor at *Yoga Journal* for a "supercool assignment that might be up your alley." "It's a story," the editor wrote, "on how the music world is bursting with yogis. We wanna talk to musicians and yogis about how both music and yoga evoke a similar feeling state, how asana can be enhanced by a great beat, and how yoga is unleashing a backstage quiet previously unheard of in the land of sex, drugs, rock 'n' roll."

The magazine thought it might be fun to get sound bytes from such paragons of rock as Sting and Edie Brickell. My friend's interest in the piece could be summed up in three words: "do not want." I, on the other hand, could see several advantages to doing a story like this. First, I'd get to do free yoga classes in places that I otherwise couldn't afford. Also, I'd be able to pay my rent. I told her to give the magazine my name.

Yoga Journal began publication in the mid-1970s, during yoga's Berkeley-and-Madison phase. In the beginning it was, like the world it covered, extremely earnest and a little dry. Over the years, as yoga evolved, so did its journal, and by the beginning of the twenty-first century, it was the full-on standard-bearer of the yoga lifestyle, putting beautiful, impossibly thin women on its cover, anointing hot new teachers, and providing extremely useful physical, mental, and relationship advice to those lucky Americans who'd discovered the yogic way.

It took a few days to persuade *Yoga Journal's* editor-in-chief that a guy who'd once recorded a song called "I Wipe My Ass on Your Novel" was the right choice to do a feature that quoted Edie Brickell. But a senior editor's enthusiasm for my previous work, however misguided, prevailed, and I got an email back saying they thought I'd do a "killer job."

Yoga had consumed my social hours, steamrolled my family life, and infiltrated my reading list. I sometimes watched yoga DVDs instead of movies at night. Sometimes, if felt as though I had space for little else in my brain. Now it was about to take over my professional life as well.

The editor sent an email elaborating on the story idea: "This feature is essentially about the intersection of asana and pop music: who and how and why are they coming together. Basically, it's a trend story about the way American yogis are building a bridge between music and yoga: classes with live music or DJs, hip-hop yoga, musicians traveling with yoga teachers on staff to keep them in a positive, flexible groove while on tour (or the famous Sting & Trudy yoga retreat in Italy)." She added that I would not, in fact, be allowed to attend that retreat.

I'd had this kind of assignment before. They obviously knew what they wanted. My job was to make the calls, attend the classes, do the required background reading, listen to the appropriate music, and deliver the goods with complete earnestness. In case you didn't read the story, it will perhaps disappoint you to learn that I did exactly what they asked, down to the final fact-check. I was a professional, and understood that this was *Yoga Journal*. Snark, attitude, or skepticism need not apply.

A feature in *Yoga Journal*, I quickly discovered, is something that many yoga professionals greatly desire. I was used to being ignored by politicians, and often found myself beaten and bowed by ruthless Hollywood publicists. Therefore, I was pretty surprised by the enthusiastic response I received when I played the *Yoga Journal* card, though perhaps I shouldn't have been. Yogis, despite their selfless reputations, are as hungry for publicity as everyone else. However, they're also much friendlier than average. Calls got returned quickly. Short emails were answered with multiple responses containing bits of wisdom and subsequent clarifications to those bits. A guy from Florida offered to fly me, all expenses paid, to his studio so I could see what he'd been doing, which turned out to be pretty much what everyone else was doing, only in Florida.

One not-at-all-self promotional yoga scholar talked to me about the Vedic tradition of *nada yoga,* the yoga of sound. *Ragas,* or devotional songs, had long been used to accompany physical yoga practice. In traditional *nada yoga,* scales were calibrated to match certain *mantras.* Now, this scholar said, yoga in the West was evolving sufficiently to incorporate music into *asana.* "There's more and more need to connect to the cultural energies of yoga, which take yoga and connect it to a mother tradition," he said. "In a way, we've been isolated here, unlike practicing in India, here we don't have a cultural energy framework. Music is a way to connect to these larger cultural energies. That's why it's making more and more of an impact." In a sure sign that I'd gone cuckoo for yoga, that quote made perfect sense to me.

Seeking a "cultural framework" for my story, I went to the West Side to interview a talented young musician who'd been playing guitar in yoga classes for several years. He got started, he said, at "conscious gatherings" in Chicago, and then answered an ad on Craigslist looking for musicians to play at something called "candlelight yoga." After a "deep meditation," he told me, he decided to move to California to pursue a career as a yoga musician.

He called guitar playing "finger asana," and said that when he's playing in class, he's practicing yoga himself. It's like "scoring a movie in real time," he said. I nodded in serious assent as he said to me, "music is the organization of the universe; it's how we perceive the harmony and dissonance in life. There are certain combinations of notes and rhythms that align with our breath and our heartwaves and brainwaves. I'm using sacred principles that trance people out. Everything is vibration."

Then he gave me a CD with an Aleph on the cover.

"Thanks for that," I said.

"So what's your angle on this story?" he said.

He'd snapped me out of my yoga trance. "Um, urgh, blergh," I said. Then I repeated, more or less verbatim, my assignment email from the magazine. Even if I wore hemp yoga pants on assignment, I was still nothing more than a journalistic whore-monkey.

Southern California was full of famous yoga teachers, millionaire wizards whose lifestyles had been lauded in the L.A. *Times* and whose DVDs adorned the shelves of boutique hotels everywhere. I'd studied with none of them. When I'd moved to town, with the promise of yoga's version of "Paris in the '20s" in my mind, I had no idea what I'd encounter. Then I moved to the East Side, twenty-five miles away from where the famous people taught, and flowed into my own life.

Though I had a wandering eye for new experience, my inherent cheapness kept me from seeking out a famous teacher at an expensive studio. Many people who went to Paris in the '20s never got anywhere near Ernest Hemingway or Gertrude Stein, and yet they still wrote, or at least thought about writing. It also had to do with L.A.'s geographical limitations. If I could walk fifteen minutes to a good yoga practice, there was no need to drive an hour and a half in traffic. I didn't even go to *restaurants* in Santa Monica, many of which were way better than the overpriced hipster dumps that my crowd tended to frequent, so why would I go to yoga studios there?

Most famous yoga teachers are famous for a reason. They have tremendous amounts of skill, wisdom, and experience to impart. But, I realized, you don't need to study with a famous teacher to learn yoga. You just need to study with a *good* one, as part of a community of friendly people. Until I got my *Yoga Journal* assignment, I'd never really felt tempted to broach the trendier districts of yoga culture. That was the first impetus for this middle-aged man to head to the West Side, toward his yoga manifest destiny.

On a sunny Monday morning (there's really no other kind of Monday morning in Los Angeles), I went to Maha Yoga, which occupies some extremely expensive real estate on the third floor of an open-air Brentwood shopping atrium. Maha is the domain of Steve Ross, a former professional guitarist who played with Fleetwood Mac, The Beach Boys, and Men at Work. Ross also trained as a monk in the Vedic tradition and toured with a guru around the United States for four years while living what he called an "intense and traditional" lifestyle, rising every day at 3 AM, meditating, chanting, doing good works, and adhering to a strict vegetarian diet. He certified as a yoga teacher in 1980, long before it was trendy, but he definitely caught the wave, and spent the next twenty years building a white-hot following of students who matter, like the yoga version of Warren Beatty's character in *Shampoo*.

In 2000, Ross debuted as the star guru of *Inhale*, the Oxygen Network's yoga show, in which he led with smarmy confidence a roomful of people better looking and more flexible than you. *Inhale*'s most notable feature—besides the brutal, bone-twisting workout you get when you practice to it—is the blaring soundtrack of cheesy pop music that accompanies every class. This became Ross' signature early on. Even though he practiced *kirtan* chanting in private, and taught weekly classes at his studio for those who were interested, he didn't think most of his students were ready. He heard them pumping loud music on their car stereos as they pulled up to class, or saw them screaming into their cell phones. These were busy Southern California trendoids. Putting them into a traditionally quiet, ascetic yoga environment, he figured, would be like unwittingly dropping them into a tub of ice water: totally jarring, and not very fun.

So he started playing music in classes. Purist yogis criticized him, saying that music in class went against tradition. Sure it's untraditional, he said, but so are blocks, straps, walls, or group classes. Traditional yoga involved fasting and living in a cave. The people who were criticizing him smoked cigars and ate meat. Who were they to deny him a little fun?

I went to class with a friend who's usually up for some yoga tourism. The yoga room was bright and spacious, like the waiting area of a prosperous independent production company. French doors opened to the north and south, letting in gentle, smoggy sea breezes. Rows of cubbies, stacked five high, occupied most of one wall, each deep enough to hold at least a couple Christian Louboutin shopping bags.

This wasn't my neighborhood studio, where ten students meant a good turnout. It filled up here. By the time we checked in, at least fifteen minutes before class, mats were already touching one another. People had lined up foot-to-nose, and everyone was doing their pre-class preening. Some rested with the help of multiple props arranged just so, indicating they were ready to fight through any level of discomfort and pain to get that special yoga feeling. Others did outrageous stretching. The real show-offs in the room performed backbends or headstands, as though what the teacher was about to put us through wouldn't be enough.

I found an open spot on the far end of the room, away from the entrance, directly under a nine-foot-high speaker propped on a tripod. My pre-class ritual began, as it always does, erratically. It was the usual mix of half-assed hip stretches, seated meditations where I mostly scratched my nose and adjusted my shorts, and a couple of minutes on my back, pretending to rest but really feeling jittery and stomach-knotty, like I'd just eaten an entire case of Junior Mints. As I lay prone, unwittingly inhaling the strong personal scent of the deliberately scruffy, handsome actor-type next to me, Steve Ross appeared in the middle of the room, as though he'd just materialized out of nowhere. He and his shaved head glided toward the stage, tall, calm, and confident.

"Everybody up!" he shouted.

He flicked on a club-quality stereo and loud synthe-sized music roared out of the speaker just above my head. This jarred me out of whatever meditative state I'd managed to achieve. The favorite music of a cool boomer began to play. We did yoga to Prince, U2, Tom Petty, and various horrific beats that usually serve as the backdrop to massive cocaine consumption. Ross cheered out the poses like a handsome, heterosexual Richard Simmons. Sweat soon slicked my brow. Moisture began to pour off my body. My sweat catcher and natural rubber mat were no match for the deluge. I was a small Midwestern town unprepared for the rising flood waters.

During seemingly endless variations on half-moon

pose, my gaze wandered. In the middle of the room were three guys, shirtless, with hairless, rippling chests. Their bodies were sleek, perfect, and fully on display. They seemed to be practicing yoga in another dimension. While the rest of us wheezed through our sequences, they were doing all kinds of crazy headstands and arm balances, slowly raising and lowering their legs with extreme control, as though a one-armed handstand was something they did during ordinary conversation. To them, yoga was a remote control, and they'd mastered the art of changing channels. They went in and out of their balances, occasionally returning to the regularly scheduled practice, then back to their super-practice, and our undying admiration.

Meanwhile, no one was wasting his or her time in class looking at me. But if they had, it would have looked like I'd gotten splashed by Shamu at Sea World; my T-shirt had uncomfortably pasted itself to my nipples. I took it off, revealing a thick, wet field of chest hair that fanned out way below my belly button. In addition, I had a big old *bindi* of a zit right in the middle of my upper chest, just along my collarbone.

So, yes, I was definitely getting a workout. Ross called for a pose that involved twisting around and clasping hands under my front leg at a near-impossible angle. This, in yoga terms, is called "binding." Well, I'd never done this particular bind before, but now, suddenly, I was doing it, and easily. I'd figured I'd get there eventually, but not necessarily to the tune of "Lady Marmalade," the Beyoncé remix.

"Voulez-vous couchez avec moi ce soir?" Beyoncé asked as Steve Ross roamed the room like a mellow, priapic deity, the Pan of yoga, winking at everyone, especially the ladies.

He went over to my friend, leaned down, and whispered in her ear, "Where have you been the last two years?"

"Definitely not here," she said.

Who were these giggly girls with their fake boobs, toe rings, and red Kabbalah strings? Why did they all seem to like this? My friend later explained that these were people who'd spent most of the last two decades doing drugs and drinking in nightclubs. Now they couldn't handle night-clubs anymore, so they were doing yoga instead. "I think I've found my people," she said to me.

Well, I never spent a lot of time in nightclubs. I wasted my youth going to indie rock concerts and poetry readings. On the East Side, the people with whom I usually practiced yoga tended toward the types who hadn't slept in three weeks because they were trying to finish their dissertation. Our music stayed in a minor key. The sex vibe was roughly equivalent to what you'd find at a Quaker Friends meeting. By comparison, walking into Steve Ross's class was like vis-iting an orgy already in progress.

During reverse warrior, I looked over at the teacher's platform. Ross was holding some hot woman's ponytail and bending her backwards until his breath was on her neck. Later, during *savasana,* I looked up again, like some kind of peeping tom. Ross kneeled in front of a particularly cute specimen, giving her a calf massage.

This guy's got sack, I thought.

At the end of class, he announced: "I'll be gone for a couple of weeks. I'm leaving tomorrow for a mental institution."

The crowd gasped. They didn't speak the language of comedy.

"Called India," he added.

After class, I sat down outside with the man that *Vanity Fair* once called "the guru of Los Angeles." Many of his students, Ross told me, were yoga teachers elsewhere in the city, but they came to his class to escape the dreary realities of the yoga world. As if to prove this point, one of the shirt-less arm-balancing studs came over. I almost didn't recognize him. He was now wearing a shirt.

"It was really awesome to come over here and feel a different vibe," he said.

After the stud left, Ross and I chatted for a while about music in yoga classes, since that, ostensibly, was my reason for being there. "Yoga should be celebratory," he told me. "That's missing in a lot of schools. I've been all over the United States to a million places. Everyone is: Push your little toe down, rotate your arm two-and-a-half degrees. That's useful as a beginner, but it's just like driving a car. Once you learn, you don't want someone in the backseat telling you how to drive. It doesn't have to be like getting slapped on the knuckles with a ruler. It doesn't have to be torture. If you watch *Inhale*, you look at how some of the people are grooving. They are *turned on*." Anyone who convincingly uses sleazy sex metaphors to describe yogic bliss is going to find a large, receptive audience in Los Angeles.

In addition to the hip-hop flow classes, he said, he also held regular weekend "ecstatic chanting" workshops, and had a CD coming out called *Give Love a Chants*. But the conversation kept veering away from music. Ross said that he'd considering writing a book of L.A. yoga gossip, called *You'll Never Do Yoga in This Town Again*. But, he said, "I want to keep teaching."

At this moment, one of his students came over and sat in his lap.

"I just want to lock him up and keep him in a box," she said as she rubbed Ross' head.

"It's been tried," he said.

Before I left, I asked him why he was going to India.

"Oh, to meditate, hang out," he said nonchalantly. "I'm friends with some monks down there."

Must be nice, I thought.

When I got home that afternoon, I had a Facebook message from Andrew the Yoga Freak, my friend from the Yogathon. He invited me to a class that he enjoyed weekly. The teacher's name was Joan, he said, and she was one of his favorites. Her Friday session at the Center for Yoga on Larchmont featured a live DJ.

"I remember you mentioning a hatred of pirates," he added, "and am wondering if you are familiar with a book titled *Sodomy and the Pirate Tradition*. It's pretty academic and dry overall, but as the title intimates, it is not without its charm. And no doubt a resource should you write about pirates and/or sodomy."

What a strange but lovely man.

In any case, a class featuring a live DJ was in my current wheelhouse, so I agreed to meet Andrew at the Center, the oldest yoga studio in Los Angeles, founded by Ganga White in 1967. It was one of the first, if not *the* first, studios in the country to take disparate *hatha* disciplines like Iyengar and Ashtanga and incorporate them into something called "flow" yoga. To make a long story as short as possible, in the 1980s, an Israeli yoga teacher named Maty Ezraty left the Center to start a studio called YogaWorks with the unfortunately named Alan Finger. YogaWorks became an influential joint, and several other studios, including Maha Yoga, were started by its most popular teachers. The founders started ramping up their business practices, unifying their teacher training with a standardized approach, asking their teachers to sign non-compete clauses, and, eventually, placing the management of the studio in the hands of an anonymous corporate "collective." They started buying up competing studios, including a very controversial 2003 purchase of the Center for Yoga, which caused a great tumult. Instructors quit in a huff, some to start their own studios. I missed the whole drama because I was, at the time, beginning my yoga practice at the Lance Armstrong 24-Hour Fitness in Austin.

Andrew had advised me to come to class early because it got crowded. It started at 4:30. I arrived at 4:05. Even if he hadn't asked me, I probably would have done that. I like to be the first guest at a party so I can sit on the couch by myself and eat chips or, in this case, stretch without bumping into other people.

The Center has several practice studios, but this class was going to be in the main salon. I peeked into the cavernous room, which had stages on two sides with a third wall taken up by wacky-looking rope contraptions. Other than the instructor and her DJ, who were setting up, Andrew was the only person in the room. He saw me, stood up from his stretching, and came over.

"I have a bunch of guest passes," he said, "or you could do this deal right now where there's a free week of yoga."

"The thing is," I said. "I'm going out of town, so I wouldn't be able to take full advantage of the free week."

He looked a bit disappointed. It didn't occur to me until later that he might have wanted to save his guest passes for other people. He took me inside and introduced me to Joan, the instructor. She said hello, then went over to the ropes, where she started hanging upside down with her ankles crossed, like Nightcrawler from the *X-Men*.

I set up next to Andrew. I'd forgotten to air out my mat after Steve Ross' class, and it didn't smell very good. The sweat catcher felt like a used washcloth after a shower. When I sat down, my mat squished with day-old sweat. This couldn't be healthy.

The practice began, and so did DJ Mattnifique. He spun some smooth grooves, exactly the kind of music I like to listen to when I'm doing yoga. Steve Ross and his cheesy 101.3 FM Jams style, while amusing, wasn't really my scene. This had a loungier feel. It was Maxwell's Urban Yoga Suite.

But my mat felt like it was deteriorating beneath my feet. It bunched up uncomfortably in weird places. I snagged my foot repeatedly on the sweat guard, and I had to break out of poses to adjust. My right wrist slipped. I barely caught myself, and I actually started to worry that I might get injured.

I got a blanket and put it over the mat, but that didn't afford me enough traction. My wrists were too close together. So now I had the additional twitchery of trying to adjust the blanket. This was the yoga equivalent of not being able to get your underwear out of your ass crack while riding the bus. You don't want to disturb the other passengers, but comfort, you know, would be nice. I looked around to see if I was bothering anyone, but Andrew was in a yoga fog, and the woman next to me didn't seem to be paying any attention to me either.

Finally, I just gave in, let the sounds of DJ Mattnifique wash over me, and made the best of the swamp mat. During a pose where I attempted to duck my head and my leg under my shoulder to do some weird airplane-type lift thing, I noticed one of the studs from Steve Ross' class doing handstands in the front row. Really, dude? What's the point of practicing in public if you're going to do that? This time, though, he was at least wearing a shirt.

Class ended. I spent most of my *savasana* having dirty sex thoughts. The *Bhagavad Gita* definitely doesn't prescribe this. But, you know, when you're totally enervated and half-asleep on a mat that feels like Ethiopian *injera* bread, your mind tends to float to primal places.

Afterward, as Andrew the Yoga Freak disappeared into the Larchmont night, I went into the lobby to talk to Joan and DJ Mattnifique. They were a couple, they told me, and had been doing these gigs together for about a year. Joan preferred live music to using an iPod. With iPods, the transitions could be rough and the songs can sometimes go five to seven minutes. A DJ can help the rhythm of the class move more seamlessly, and the teacher and DJ can read each other. It's kind of a Friday night happy-hour approach to yoga, they said.

DJ Mattnifique played a lot of private parties and had a regular weekend gig at the bar at the Sofitel, but he preferred yoga DJing. "It pays me in the real way," he said. Also, he added, "The people are a lot cooler in yoga. They're not coming up to me and burping in my face with their alcohol breath."

He explained how he liked to work a yoga class.

"What I try to do," said DJ Matt, "is in the first quarter, try to take it real nice and slow, and then in the second quarter, I crank it up high. The third quarter is a little bit of a cool down, and the . . ."

"Does everything have to be a football metaphor for you?" Joan said, teasingly, causing her partner to blush.

"And in the fourth, you really pound it home and run out the clock?" I asked.

"Not like my Eagles," he said. "They got a little running back."

"Westbrook's pretty versatile," I said. "But he goes out of bounds too much. They need a bull like LenDale White."

"This man knows his football," said DJ Matt.

"Yeah, I'm not one of these yoga hippies," I said. "I'm a real man."

"Well, all right," Matt said.

"In fact," I said, "sometimes I think about fantasy football roster moves during *savasana*. It's a really good time to make decisions."

They looked distressed. Clearly, I'd taken the male bonding too far and overstayed my interview. I put on my shoes and left sheepishly.

When I got home, I put my sweat guard in the laundry and took my mat outside for a hose-down. The next morning, on the way back to my bedroom from the shower, I found myself drifting spontaneously into warrior three, just because I could.

But as I reached the full expression of the pose in the narrow hallway, there was a quick, stabbing pain on the arch side of my left foot, just above the heel. I remembered slipping there the night before when the blanket was covering my mat. Before I took another step, I knew I was headed for injured reserve. DJ Mattnifique would have been proud.

The side of my ankle practically glowed red, and it throbbed. I iced and heated and elevated. But the foot still hurt, a lot. In a panic, I called my doctor. It was a weekend, but he returned my call and asked me to describe the injury.

"Well," I said, "it's kind of under the bone on the big toe side of the ankle, but it's not the Achilles tendon. Maybe the peroneal tendon? I don't know. I looked it up on Wikipedia. Walking's not too hard, but when I flex my foot in a certain way, or bend over, or reach up my arm, it really hurts, and . . ."

"Sounds like you have a pulled muscle," he said.

On Monday, I underwent the usual treatment regime of X-ray, cold-laser therapy, and chiropractic adjustment, which I began to suspect is what I'd have gotten even if I'd staggered into the office with an arm severed at the elbow. The X-ray revealed nothing. My diagnosis of pulled muscle got downgraded to strained tendon.

In the annals of sports injury, working through a "strained tendon from practicing on a yoga mat soggy from being left rolled up overnight" doesn't quite reach Curt Schilling bloody sock territory. Still, I had to stop practicing. It had been a long time since I'd gone more than a few days without yoga. My body didn't really notice, but my mental and emotional state began to decline. I found myself getting irritated, upset, and depressed. Self-doubt crept in. Suddenly, the littlest things began to strike me as disastrous.

One evening, I asked Regina, "Why was today so horrible?"

"It was the same as every other day," she said. "You're just losing your yoga brain."

Couldn't I have kept my yoga brain, at least for a little while, without the physical practice? I'd done all this work toward creating a better version of myself, and it was crumbling away because I had a little foot ouchie? That just wasn't fair.

"But I don't *want* to lose my yoga brain!" I moaned. "How did this happen to me?"

Actually, I knew exactly how. For the first time in my life, I had genuine strength, agility, and balance, things that had previously been present only in trace amounts. But this had happened over many years, after hundreds of long, slow, deliberate classes. Then, when I got my assignment, I started doing fast flow classes, pretty much every day. I found myself in crowded, high-octane environments, and I got nervous. I felt desperate to keep pace. Because of that, I lost focus. My alignment broke down. I'd been doing the wrong thing, and it didn't take long for my body to let me know. Still, I had to finish the *Yoga Journal* gig. There were many more classes to attend, whether I could practice in them or not.

It was 2 PM on a Saturday. Regina had gone out for coffee with a friend. I sat in my basement, watching an episode of *The IT Crowd* (the British one) on Dailymotion. Elijah lay in bed, moaning because something he'd eaten had given him gas.

There was a knock. The dogs barked. Elijah screamed, "SOMEONE IS HERE! I CAN'T GET UP BECAUSE OF MY FARTS!" I lurched up the stairs in a brown sweatshirt streaked with egg-yolk stains, my hair was sticking straight up, and I smelled worse than I looked.

By contrast, the woman standing at my door was pretty, young, tan, composed, muscular, and sleek. She held a gift bag from the Exhale Center for Sacred Movement, in Venice. I assumed this was Micheline Berry, the yoga teacher whose class I was supposed to attend the next morning as part of my assignment. She'd wanted me to have some DVDs of her yoga program, Liquid Asana, so I'd know what to expect. Also, she was throwing in some recordings from her band, Shaman's Dream, which would be playing in her class.

I extended a sweaty hand.

"Nice to meet you, Micheline," I said.

"Oh, I'm not Micheline," said the woman. "I'm her assistant."

"Yoga teachers have assistants?" I said.

"Some of them do."

"Oh."

The assistant handed me the bag, and I thanked her.

"Are you going to be in class tomorrow?" I said.

She nodded.

"I'm coming," I said, "but I don't think I'm going to be able to practice."

I pointed to my left foot, which was wrapped in an ACE bandage gone black with grime.

She looked at me kind of sympathetically.

"Yes," she said. "I read the email you sent us. It was very long. But you should come some other time. It's really an amazing practice."

I looked in the bag. The three DVDs all had Berry on the cover, looking serene and gorgeous in brightly colored unitards.

She'd written me a personal note. Mostly, it was just a

reminder of the time and address of the class. But she also said, "have a blessed day." Grumble grumble. Blessed day, my stinky butt. Why were yoga people always so goddamn nice?

The Exhale Center for Sacred Movement in Venice was exactly the kind of place I didn't practice yoga, all high ceilings and virgin-white walls. They served excellent tea and had a couch area that wouldn't have been out of place at a high-end spa. Good lord, this place was nice. Everywhere I looked, there were large, glossy posters bearing the visages of some of the center's most revered teachers. Every month, every weekend, every *day*, it seemed, they offered teacher training or special events that went far beyond what most other studios served up.

Part Two of Saul David Raye's Ecstatic Embodiment Training in the Fire Module provided one hundred hours of instruction for just $1100. A Ritual Flow of Yoga Immersion workshop, with a guest Tantric-Vedic Priest, could be yours for only $250 plus a materials fee. Advanced Pranafication Teacher Training: Tending the Fire—The Art of Living Yoga Sadhana was another $1100. No wonder the studio looked so fancy! There was also The Art of Thai Massage, Yoga And Walking, From Drama to Dharma—Be in the Flow of Prosperity Without the Fear of Scarcity, Yoga For Hormones, a few record-release parties, a handful of workshops to help with breathing techniques and to heal back pain, and Heart on Fire: An Exploration in Mind-Body Yoga and Contemporary Spirituality. What was it with these people and "hearts" and "fire"? The only time my heart caught fire was after eating a Double-Double from In-N-Out Burger.

I arrived for class early, while the musicians were setting up their instruments, including something called a *batajon*, a West African instrument otherwise known as the "fat congas." A guy in dreadlocks had brought a four-year-old boy. At one point early in the class, I looked up and saw him teaching the kid how to whack sticks together in rhythm, and I felt like a bad father. *My* son was at home watching a *Ben 10: Alien Force* marathon on Cartoon Network. But then later the kid started whining and the dad had to leave the jam early, so I felt better.

These guys were some of the members of Shaman's Dream, Micheline Berry's house yoga band. The group started, Berry told me later, when a musician named Craig Kohland attended a "zen dancing" class that she was giving in 1997. He loved it so much that he brought his drums the next time. They formed a band together, started leading "ecstatic dance journeys," and, in 2000, began accompanying classes at YogaWorks. The idea, she said, was to work with top-flight musicians, experienced improvisers, with the goal of achieving a moment of transcendence where musician and yogi disappeared into a common ecstasy of breath and movement. Sometimes they placed Tibetan bowls on people's bodies during *savasana* because the vibration creates an altered state of consciousness.

I put my mat close to the stage, so I could get an uninterrupted view of the musicians. The room filled up quickly. Just before class started, a guy slid into the space just in front of me. I hadn't thought there'd be room, but experienced practitioners are excellent at playing mat Tetris. It was a longhaired dude wearing a burnt-orange cotton pancho. *Fucking hippie,* I thought. Then his pancho came off, and I had to look at his bare back, the disgusting yellow soles of his feet, and the gray boxers that said HBO on the band that were peeking up from his yoga shorts. Perhaps I'd been too quick to judge.

Berry appeared just before class started, looking resplendent in a bright-orange top and electric yellow pants. These are not colors most people can pull off, but this woman had a fine tan. She would have looked good wearing a bulk-rice sack. Those superficialities aside, she faced quite a challenge: Leading a ninety-person class while also keeping a music ensemble in line. "It's a lot to pull together," she later admitted to me.

The music started slowly, almost imperceptibly, but by the third pose, *virasana* (or hero), the jam was in full session. Berry moved us through deliberately, sensually. I found myself thinking that this is how I liked to practice, though I would have preferred it without a rich hippie sticking his foot in my face. That said, I *wasn't* practicing, not really. I did a few lame *vinyasas* with my bad foot in the air, but then I had to back off; I couldn't do a single standing pose. Mostly, I sat on my mat, staring at my dirty bandage.

"Feel the music," Berry said. "In every last way, your body is responding to it. So in that way, *you're also making the music.*"

She told the class to start moving. I sat and watched as everyone swayed from side to side, shaking out his or her hands a little. The music picked up, and soon there was much shaking and dancing in the room.

"WHAT ARE YOU SHAKING LOOSE THIS MORNING?" Berry shouted into her wireless headset. "LET IT GO!"

She turned to the band, indicating to them with hand

gestures that the drums needed to get deeper and more intense. They obliged. The class began to go crazy, and suddenly I was sitting in the middle of some sort of Burning Man drum circle.

"WEEEEEEEE-OOOOOOOOOH!" Berry yelped.

"WEEEEEEEE-OOOOOOOOOH!" the class responded.

"You all have a wild creative intelligence that makes children, that makes marriages, that paints, that writes books, that works behind the counter, there is this *wild love* inside you that endures so much suffering . . ."

I don't know, I thought. *Most of the people in here look OK to me.*

"And I want you to think about what are you going to give this love to today. Who? *What* are you healing?"

She waved her hand. The music stopped, and the class applauded, whooped, and whistled. "Crazy!" shouted the guy in front of me.

After this all subsided, the band descended into a slow blues jam. I later learned from Berry that they'd decided to add the blues number while drinking at a party the night before. This earned my respect. She had the class do "spiral circles." Since this was a seated pose, I was able to participate.

"Feel that old river inside," she said.

The HBO hippie in front of me moaned "mmmmm-mmm," like he was on a Robert Johnson 78. At the front of the room, Berry slinked forward from the floor, into a beautiful upward-facing dog. She said,

"Rise out of the bayou . . . of your pelvis."

This, I thought, *was the single greatest instruction I'd ever heard in a yoga class.* A guy in the band sang, "You've

got to move/you've got to move/you've got to move child/
you've got to move/When the Lord/Gets ready/You've got
to move." It should have been easy to mock, but the musicians were really good. The blues ended. Berry started up
again.

"Before Zoloft, before Paxil, before Prozac, before St.
John's Wort, before Freud, Jung, Lacan, The Forum, there
was *rhythm*," she said. "It was the way we saw ourselves, the
way we continue to see ourselves. Where does this heart-
beat come from? Where does the breath come from? We
become so involved with our urban lives full of hip cynicism that we forget we are magical, mystical beings. Each
and every one of you."

Yeah, right, I thought.

The music got louder and more intense. She started
playing a noisemaker. The class swayed back and forth. I
followed along, cross-legged, on my mat.

"Feel that energy rising," she said.

The energy rose. A frenzy overtook the class. And then
the music stopped.

"Two, three, four . . ." she said.

The music started again, now really frenzied. Then
Berry went behind the stage and produced two sparkling
hula hoops. She handed these to a beautiful woman at
the front of the room, who stood up and started twirling
around. In L.A., a sexy gamine willing to do hula-hoop
stunts is never more than a phone call away. The woman
whipped them up and down her body, on her neck, on her
arms, on her outstretched legs, all while keeping time to the
music. The crowd lost its rhythm and started watching her
instead. Oh, she was mesmerizing. But now the yoga was a

Vegas floor show, a circus. What came next, fire jugglers? The woman bent up and down and all around, the center of attention, a state to which she appeared quite accustomed.

When it was over, the class whooped and applauded. I realized that this is what the rest of the world probably thinks Southern California is like all the time.

"This is why I teach in Venice," the teacher said. "I couldn't get away with this anywhere else."

I was back at the Center for Yoga, interviewing a musician from a three piece ensemble that sometimes accompanies classes there. She had an instrument called a *hang*, a highly intellectualized variation on the steel drum. In 2000, a couple of Swiss guys invented the *hang* in Bern. There are, the musician told me, only five thousand *hangs* in existence, and only seven people in California play them. "People only sell them when they have financial difficulties, or if they don't know what they have," she said. "They're actually considered a sound sculpture." The new version, for 2009, was called the *integral hang*, and it only played one note. She didn't have an integral *hang*. Hers bore nine indentations, which, when deployed properly, hit all the "vibrational chakras." It wasn't invented for yoga specifically, but adapted easily to the practice.

"When I play any instrument," she said, "my intention is to channel the divine."

Eventually, as in most of my conversations, we started talking about me, in particular all the live-music-yoga experiences I'd had recently. At some point, I mentioned Steve Ross.

"Oh, yeah," said one of the musicians. "That was the guy who was held hostage in Mumbai."

"What?" I said. "Are you sure?"

"Pretty sure," he said.

Then I remembered that I'd received an email from Maha Yoga, "gratefully welcoming" Steve back from his trip to Mumbai. "Join us for a beautiful evening of chanting guaranteed to open your heart," it read. I'd deleted it immediately.

When I got home, I found Maha Yoga's Facebook page. There were a few status updates from the past week. The first read: "Thank you to all who have inquired as to Steve Ross' safety while he is in Mumbai. We have confirmed information that Steve is safe in his hotel under the protection of military and police. We do not have any further details at this time but will do our best to update this site with news on his welfare and return to Los Angeles as soon as information is available. In the meantime, please send your prayers to all those involved in this tragic situation."

Wow, I thought. He hadn't just happened to be in Mumbai at the time of the attacks. He'd been at the *center* of the action. The next update read:

"Steve is perfectly fine and calm. He was so touched that everyone was concerned about him. He is comfortable and planning to return to L.A. in a couple of days."

Next to that was a link to a video that showed the release of hostages from the Oberoi Hotel. There was Ross, looking very happy to be free as he walked out of the hotel's front door. Maha later posted this on their website: "We are very happy to announce that Steve Ross and his group have been evacuated from the Oberoi Hotel. Our prayers go out to all those involved and especially to the family of Steve's friends Alan and Naomi Scherr who lost their lives during these tragic events. Steve will return to Los Angeles at the end of next week. With love—Maha Yoga."

So Steve had been friends with two of the victims. *How horrible for him,* I thought, *but what a story!* Master yoga teacher and television star goes to India to meditate with monks, but instead is taken hostage by terrorists with ties to al-Queda. The only place this had been covered was a blog called The Accidental Yogist, which focused on the L.A. scene. They'd done one post, which had received zero comments. No other media outlet had touched the story. I, on the other hand, had attended Ross' final yoga class before he'd left for India. In fact, I was probably the last person to interview him, and I had scenes of him acting calm and comfortable, lightly flirting with his students, a man at the top of his profession with not a care in the world, which would give the story even extra depth.

Once again the worst version of myself began to take over my brain. I was consumed by careerist dreams and visions of glory. *This was the yoga story of the century,* I thought, *and it was all mine.* I'd report the hell out of the piece, publish it somewhere, and win multiple local-press prizes, maybe even a National Magazine Award nomination. It would get optioned, and maybe I'd get first crack at the screenplay. I felt like a yoga version of Kirk Douglas' character in *Ace in the Hole,* conveniently forgetting that Douglas ended the movie dead on the newsroom floor from a stab wound.

I called Maha Yoga. A woman answered the phone.

"Hi," I said. "This is Neal Pollack. I interviewed Steve for *Yoga Journal* before he left for Mumbai."

"Hi, Neal," she said flatly.

"Anyway, I heard about what happened to him. How terrible. Is he OK?"

"He's fine."

Even flatter.

"So, listen, this may not be appropriate, but . . ."

"Steve has told us not to talk to the press," she said.

"But will *he* talk?" I asked.

"He's said he doesn't want to do any press. Not for any reason. Not even for healing."

"Not even for healing?"

"No."

"Huh," I said.

In my mind, I searched for a strategy, an in, some sort of angle. But when the person about whom you want to write a story refuses to talk to the press, that story's pretty much shut down. *Perhaps,* I thought, *this was for the best.* My overambitious thoughts had done nothing but distract me from the true yogi's path. I'd just take my *Yoga Journal* assignment, be satisfied with it, and not try to push my yoga reportage any further. Goddamn it.

"Well then," I said, "I'll just let you go!"

She said that Steve would be chanting that Friday night, and I was welcome to come celebrate with all his other students.

"Oh," I said, "thank you so much."

But I was thinking, *Please, who the hell wants to haul out to Brentwood on a Friday afternoon?*

10

Bikram Begins

For months, every time I'd driven past the Bikram studio on Glendale Boulevard, I'd felt guilty. The ultimate opportunity for supreme mental clarity and physical fitness was right there, walking distance of my house if I didn't mind choking on the truck fumes from I-5. They had a deal where you could take classes for seven consecutive days for only twenty bucks. I was running out of excuses, but the thought of Bikram made me very nervous; I tended to sweat a lot just taking the trashcans down to the end of the driveway. If I did twenty-six yoga poses twice over in a room heated to 105 degrees, I would be like the Ganges during monsoon season. Finally, though, a few weeks after filing my piece for *Yoga Journal*, I decided it was time to try Bikram.

"You'll be fine," a wise yoga friend said to me. "Don't push yourself too hard and don't be competitive with everyone who's going agro around you."

"Oh, I won't," I said. "Agro is rarely my problem."

The night before my first Bikram class, I got my stretchy shorts out of the drawer where I kept all my yoga clothes. I gave the shorts a sniff. Now I knew what a month's worth of ass smelled like.

"I need to wash these," I said to my wife.

"They're gonna smell a lot worse than that tomorrow," Regina said.

Regina, in general, was tired of my relentless yoga-ing, but she had a particularly strong bias against Bikram. This stemmed from the time when she was driving past the studio in Atwater Village and she saw a woman emerge from the front door, kneel on the sidewalk, and yarf the full contents of her stomach into the gutter. At that moment, Regina determined that she would never ever do Bikram Yoga, not ever until the end of time, not even under the penalty of death, not even if doing Bikram were a mandatory qualification for watching the series finale of *Battlestar Galactica*. She was more likely to disembowel a puppy by hand or feign interest in my fantasy baseball team. Nevertheless, she attempted to muster a faint wisp of sympathetic support for my misguided desires. An hour before my class, she handed me something.

"Here," she said. "Take Elijah's towel."

"It's dirty," I said.

"It's not dirty. Those are fingerprints."

"Then what's this brown stain? I am not taking an ass towel to Bikram."

She gave it a sniff.

"That's not ass. It's food."

Never mind why our son was drying himself with a food-stained towel. This wasn't coming to class with me.

"No," I said.

"I am *not* going to sacrifice one of our good towels," she said. "For this . . . for this *thing*."

"I'm just going to sweat," I said. "There'll be no sacrifice."

Regina went into the bathroom.

"What are you doing?" I said.

"I'm tearing apart our linen closet looking for a towel for you to take to your stupid yoga class."

"But I have to pee!" I said.

"Tough!" I really did have to pee. So I went to the backyard and watered my favorite tree. When I returned, she'd chosen a towel. Like Elijah's food towel, it was also white.

"Is this the same towel?" I asked.

"No, it's not. Now go do your yoga, asswipe."

I arrived early to find the door locked. So I sat on the planter outside for a while, until a bearded dude wearing a hoodie crossed the street. He let me inside. There wasn't much there except changing rooms and a bunch of pamphlets extolling the many virtues of Bikram Yoga. I crinkled through the papers. A woman, wearing a tank top and what appeared to be a shiny black diaper, zipped out of the adjacent studio.

"Can I help you with something?" she said.

"I'm here for the eleven-thirty," I said.

"Have a seat," she said, pointing to a bench. "And sit very, very still."

There I remained, alone, for ten minutes, until a mousy dude wearing thick glasses appeared. He was a Bikram devotee. I was lucky to be beginning my practice in Atwater, he said. The teachers here were very nice. They could get kind of hard-core at other places.

When my teacher finally appeared (she'd been taking the earlier class), I filled out a little form, gave her my twenty bucks, and went inside. Yep, it was hot in there all right, a carpeted hell-sauna. The room had floor-to-ceiling mirrors on three sides. There were hallways on either end of the rear wall, leading to unisex bathrooms. In between hung two glossy portraits of a man, forehead exposed but hair shoulder-length in the back. In one of them, he wore a loincloth and sat atop a rug bearing a snarling tiger's head. This was Bikram Choudhury, the reason I was placing my mat on a sisal carpet, taking care to align the upper left corner on the little blue dot. These dots were evenly dispersed around the room to make sure that everyone had adequate personal space in which to faint.

The teacher asked if anyone was a first-timer. Only I raised my hand. She told me to take it easy if I wanted.

"Not a problem," I said.

I got through the breathing exercises and initial postures without too much trouble. In fact, I wasn't even sweating that much. I'd sweated more in flow classes. This was going to be fine.

Suddenly, I began to feel a little woozy. As I rose up from a tough crouching posture, I saw black spots in front of my eyes. For a second, my vision went black. A massive wave of nausea overwhelmed me. I imagined running into the bathroom and unleashing my guts into the toilet, and thought about how awesome that would feel.

I dropped to my hands and knees.

"Ohhhhhh," I said.

The instructor came over.

"Have you got water?" she said.

I pointed toward my little sixteen-ounce Sigg bottle, made from authentic recycled Swedish aluminum.

"That's not enough," she said.

She left the room as we rested between poses, and came back with a big plastic bottle of clear, cold water.

"Take little sips," she said.

"Right," I said, and took three huge gulps.

From there, I endured. I didn't do all the postures, but the practice got a lot easier once the standing poses ended. As my mind cleared and my stomach relaxed, my awesome powers of observation returned.

For instance, I noticed that the teacher peppered her class with a lot of foreign-language terms, and they weren't Sanskrit. For instance, before doing a pose, she'd say *prego*, and then between poses, instead of "change," she'd say "*changer*," as in the French pronunciation *shawn-jay*. She also sermonized mildly as I dripped sweat all over myself. Apparently, her brother, a "gym guy," had been getting bored with his routine. She'd been trying to get him to come to yoga for years, but he refused because he was afraid of yoga.

"But you can't be afraid," she said. "You just have to come to yoga."

Exactly, I thought, as I dipped in and out of consciousness.

Finally, mercifully, the class ended. The instructor turned to me and said "How about a big hand for our friend Neal here?"

There was mild applause.

"I guess it's safe now to tell you that the room was 112 degrees today," she said.

"What?"

It was only supposed to be 105 degrees. Sometimes, the teacher said, they turn up the heat in dry climates. *That's it,* I thought. *I'm moving to Portland.*

I returned home.

"How was it?" Regina said.

"Horrible."

"How do you feel?"

"Lightheaded. Calm. Tired. Everything looks fuzzy around the edges."

"Dude, your face is totally red."

"Am I glowing?"

"Just red."

"I have a fucking headache."

"Put those shorts in the wash, right now."

"They're fine."

"No, they're not."

I went to sleep at midnight, but by 4:30 AM, I was awake again. My brain felt scrambled. Bikram had fucked with my head. Not since I'd first started taking Wellbutrin had my thoughts been shuffled in quite this way. Over a long weekend, the drug had caused me to relive my entire life backwards while causing my heart to pound at three times its normal speed. That's about where I was after one day of Bikram, except that this time, the muscles in my left bicep and right calf wouldn't stop twitching.

All morning, I teetered between sleep and wakefulness. I spent an hour in bed, an hour at my desk, and back and forth again. Finally, at 10 AM, my day officially began. *Fuck it,* I thought, as I got out of bed for the last time. I'd paid for seven days of Bikram. I was going to get my money's worth.

"I'm going back," I said to Regina.

"For a second day in a row?" she asked. "Is that wise?"

"Probably not," I said.

But I felt almost hypnotized. Despite my mental and physical misery, I wanted to go back to the studio. It called to me, like a ghost across the moor seeking its long-ago-forbidden love. Maybe the Bikram people had put something in my water, and were turning me into a yoga zombie.

I got to the studio early, again, and soon I was on my mat feeling not so bad, stamina-wise. There was no nausea, only a little dizziness and a lingering feeling of strange. Bikram poses had different alignments than what I was used to; the flow seemed off to me. Plus, because of the heat, I found myself pushing further into poses than I wanted, and certainly more than was necessary.

Three poses in, the right side of my lower back locked up. My spine felt stiff and raw. Someone, possibly Bikram himself, was metaphorically stabbing my lumbar vertebrae with a knife.

I called the instructor over.

"Um," I said. "My lower back."

"Do you have a herniated disc?" she said.

"Christ, I hope not."

"Or did you just strain something?"

"Yeah, that."

"No sit-ups," she said. *Not a problem,* I thought. "And be very careful with the forward folds."

A tube of Arnica appeared in her hand.

"This stuff helps," she said.

I arched backward and smeared stuff on the bad area. Rivulets of sweat shot up my nose. When I was done, the teacher spread a towel on my back and sat on me, hard. Man, did that feel good. But my back throbbed for the rest of the class, certainly too much for me to enjoy *savasana.*

When it was all over, I sat cross-legged, looking at myself in the front-wall mirror. A gray shadow seemed to descend over my body. Then, slowly, as if I were undergoing a corporeal eclipse, it appeared, at least to me, that my face began to turn black. The blackness creeped down my neck, and then my torso, and beyond, until I only saw myself in the mirror in black outline, as though there were a void, in the shape of my body, where I'd been sitting.

This was what bothered me about Bikram Yoga. You spent the whole practice gazing in the mirror. Your muscles strained, your body glistened, and you got to admire yourself the whole time. But from what I understood about yoga philosophy, the whole point was to separate from your self, *not* to notice your body. By looking at myself in the mirror, I was over-acknowledging the fact that I was doing yoga. It seemed self-absorbed, cultish, and horrible. My soul felt like it was rotting, not lifting up toward something higher. I'd woken in the middle of the night with an unquenchable desire to do Bikram again. That wasn't normal. It was a sign of evil.

I hobbled back to my car. My torso had shifted to the left, and was no longer aligned with my hips. Fifteen more minutes of Bikram Yoga, and it probably would have detached itself entirely. For five days, I dragged the right side of my body beside me like a useless pseudopod. Eventually, it got better, *because I wasn't doing yoga.*

The Legend of Bikram goes as follows: Born in Calcutta in 1946, Bikram Choudhury began studying yoga at the age of four with Bishnu Charan Ghosh, brother of Paramahansa Yogananda, author of *Autobiography of a Yogi.* He practiced four to six hours a day at Ghosh's Center for Physical Culture, and, at age eleven, became the youngest-ever winner of the National India Yoga Championship. According to Bikram—every known fact about Bikram comes straight from his own mouth, including the fact that Elvis Presley was his "best friend" in the 1970s—he won the title three consecutive years until Bishnu Ghosh asked him to retire to give other competitors a chance. The great Swami Sivananda declared Bikram "Yogi Raj," King of the Yogis, and Bikram's work, it seemed, was done.

From there, Bikram became a marathon runner and a champion weightlifter, representing India in the 1964 Olympics in Tokyo. In 1966, a possibly apocryphal "weightlifting accident" left twenty-year-old Bikram crippled. Doctors told him he'd never walk again. So he returned to his guru. Together, they developed what became Bikram's twenty-six-pose series, and Bikram found himself fully healed and able to open yoga schools throughout Asia.

Bikram told the following story on *60 Minutes*, so it must be true: In 1972 President Richard Nixon suffered an attack of phlebitis while visiting the South Pacific. The President's doctor summoned Bikram and begged him to give Nixon the full hot-yoga treatment. On *60 Minutes,* Bikram said: "He got up, shave, with the dress, tie, suit, went for meeting. And he asked me first thing, 'Sir, who are you? Are you an Indian black magician?'" Bikram explained that he was a yogi. Nixon then personally invited him to come and live in the United States.

A year later, Bikram arrived on America shores, and began a thirty-five-year march toward total market domination. Along the way, he decided that every Bikram studio should teach the same poses in the same order, in the same way, everywhere in the world. When people started calling Bikram Yoga "McYoga," he ran with the comparison: "What's wrong with that? I eat Big Mac. That means, they mean, correct me if I'm wrong, it's getting more popular. You know, spreading out all over like McDonald's."

Bikram soon began suing his competition, or, as he put it, "defending my spirit, sweat, blood and tears." In the early 2000s, he began sending cease-and-desist letters to studios that were teaching something other than his exact method under the name "Bikram Yoga." This led to lawsuits and counter-suits, but Bikram emerged victorious, when a federal judge ruled that a yoga sequence, like a song or the dance steps in a ballet, may be copyrighted. "Yoga belongs to the earth," Bikram said. "It's a god. But I picked up a piece of it and I created something."

Bikram once famously told *Business 2.0* magazine that his yoga was the "only yoga." Asked why, he said it was because he has "balls like atom bombs, two of them, 100 megatons each. Nobody fucks with me." This statement, albeit quite awesome, didn't really explain why Bikram was the "only yoga." But because Bikram is prone to saying such things, other yoga circles view him and his particular craft with everything from mildly dismissive amusement to a disdain verging on disgust. Bikram is determined to get competitive yoga added to the Summer Olympics. He's having a hard time persuading non-Bikram people to join him. But with atomic testicles, he may not need their help.

To people like myself who've spent years practicing yoga in an atmosphere of soft-lit candles, chanting, and nonjudgmental good vibes, the idea of a yoga competition sounds about as absurd as the idea of competitive prayer. But I was a yoga reporter now, and in February 2009, I got an assignment from Slate.com to cover the Sixth Annual International Yoga Asana Championship. On my way to the traditional yoga setting of the Westin LAX, I steeled myself for some sort of whacked-out yoga circus, and that's more or less what I got. But a lot of yoga culture felt weird and circus-like to me anyway. I would have been disappointed if it had ended up being otherwise.

At the center of the weekend, wearing flashy suits and various fedoras, stood Bikram Choudhury. In the yoga world, only Bikram would have the chutzpah, at the opening ceremony of a rigorous athletic event, to throw himself a lavish birthday party (funded by his affiliate-studio owners) in an enormous hotel ballroom appointed like the dining room of a middlebrow cruise ship. The evening's program, a nonstop cavalcade of Bikram worship that flowed like a river of artificially sweetened ghee, included: an enthusiastic performance from the Bikram-yoga-practicing dance team Pepe and the Outer Circle Crew; a confused presentation from Ogie the Wild Man, a Bikram devotee also known as "the world's fastest golfer"; and a performance of the Shirley Horn song "Here's to Life," with lyrics changed: *Here's to life, to every joy it brings/here's to life, to Bikram and his dreams.*

The evening ended with Bikram giving a short birthday speech about the economic crisis. Life is like waves in the ocean, he said: one up, one down. You have to stay afloat as long as possible until the waves hit the beach, and yoga is the only thing that can keep you going for certain. "Every business is going down," Bikram said. "But yoga is going up sixty percent." By the end, Bikram was onstage with Pepe and the Outer Circle Crew, wearing a red, spangled shirt and out-dancing everyone to a disco remix of "Sweet Dreams (Are Made of This)." *Well,* I thought, *at least someone is having a good year.*

When I returned the next morning, the room had been transformed into a legitimate athletic stage, with no evidence of the previous night's variety-show nuttiness save a few stray balloons in the rafters. Everything ran with precision and efficiency. The video and audio were of professional quality and the emcee had a classy, sonorous voice. Most impressive, the competitors, judged under strict and consistent standards, continually flowed into beautiful and magnificent yoga postures.

The men were all more than competent. But watching the women was like staring at water slowly being poured from a pitcher. They were lyrical, majestic, composed. Legs folded behind heads, and heads appeared between legs, chin on the floor, after impossible backward bends. Yoginis would fold into lotus, balance on their knees, and shoot their legs back while balancing on their arms, smiling the whole time. I may have been dreaming but I swear I saw, during the youth competition, one girl draw into a bow, arch back, and place her toes in her mouth. I'd been doing yoga for years, but this was the first time I'd seen poses performed like this. They looked like the fakirs I used to gawk at in the Guinness Book of World Records. What they did may not have been Olympian, but it was quite a feat.

Yoga competitions have a long and respected tradition in India. Bikram's wife, Rajashree, is also a legendary champion. When I talked to her between events in the ballroom, she remembered how, at the time she married Bikram in 1984, India was lobbying to get yoga into the Olympics. That attempt went nowhere, since at the time no other country had enough skilled yogis to field a team.

Even in 2003, when Bikram and Rajashree held their first tournament to honor Bishnu Ghosh's centenary, the field included only the United States, India, Canada, and Australia; men and women competed against one another directly. But this year's field featured competitors from twenty countries (still not enough to qualify for the Olympics), with separate men's and women's divisions, as well as competitions for boys and girls under the age of eighteen. There are well-attended regional competitions throughout the year featuring yogis from nearly every American state.

While the wave is clearly rising, it's still far from megacorporate status. This year's "official sponsors" were a few yoga-wear companies, most of them owned by Bikram people, and Zico coconut water. Still, Bikram's global reach, ambition, resources, and a bull-dogged marketing scheme were enough to draw several members of the International Olympic Committee to the Westin. "Everything has to happen at the right time," Rajashree told me confidently. "This is the right time."

The end goal of all yoga is to get to *dharma-megha samadi*, a state of enlightened bliss where the ego separates from the self and the practitioner realizes that he's powerless to control the vagaries of an endlessly shifting universe. Obviously, this can't be quantified. Instead, yoga competitions involve various asanas, or poses, within *hatha*, the physical branch of yoga. As in diving, figure skating, or Platonic philosophy, there's an ideal form.

The basic competition involves five compulsory poses: standing-head-to-knee, which looks just like it sounds; standing bow, in which you balance on one leg with one arm extended forward and the other arm drawing back the lifted leg; bow pose, in which, sitting on the floor, you grab both feet with your hands and arch back; "rabbit," which involves scrunching up into a little ball; and a seated forward stretch. After that, the competitors get to pick two optional poses, where they can really strut. They have three minutes to complete the routine.

On Saturday afternoon, I met Mary Jarvis, a San Francisco-based yoga-studio owner who was one of Bikram's first American students. She's kind of like the Béla Kårolyi of competitive yoga; she's trained several world champions and several more runners-up. Jarvis walked me through the basics of the competition with a refreshing bluntness. The first two poses, she said, are about patience, strength, and endurance, while the seated poses are purely biomechanical and reveal the quality of your spine. Your optional poses "tell a story about the kind of person you are," she said. "You demonstrate what you've accomplished in your life. It's brilliant. You cannot lie."

Competitive yoga, Jarvis told me, is about the unity of body, mind, and soul. "The more advanced a yoga posture is, the more humble the yogi should be," she said. "If somebody's really arrogant, I won't train them. They can have a great posture on stage and be a total asshole."

To a hard-core yoga dork like myself, explanations like hers make sense. Yoga had done more for my physical and mental well-being than anything else I'd tried. Still, I didn't regularly practice Bikram Yoga, and that's where, as the competitions entered their final hours on Sunday, my problems with the whole thing lay.

In order to make competitive yoga Olympics-worthy, Rajashree had started a not-for-profit federation. She was acting, she said, as an objective ambassador of yoga, and anybody from any discipline was welcome to compete in these championships. This seemed like a worthy sentiment, and an evidently sincere one, except that those outreach efforts didn't appear to be going anywhere. Every single person I met at the Westin was a Bikram teacher, student, or studio owner, and they all described their experience with Bikram while wearing the eye-glaze of the recently saved. All the postures in the compulsory series are drawn from Bikram's copyrighted practice, as were nearly all the optional poses I saw.

When I mentioned my own baseline yoga practice, the Ashtanga primary series, I was met with a quiet nod of silent judgment or a dismissive "hmm." One person said, "Well, if you want to go practice your *ujayii* breath off in the corner, that's your business." In this, they take their lead from their guru, who in a recent interview said that prop-heavy Iyengar yoga studios look like "a Santa Monica sex shop."

Though I didn't quite feel that my kind were welcome, I did admire the dedication and hard training of the athletes. Every competitor I met took the hot, brutal punishment of Bikram Yoga at least once a day; that regimen, as well as extra practice time, would suck the life out of just about anyone. I talked with twenty-three-year-old Joseph Encinia of Dallas, who four years earlier had been an overweight kid with rheumatoid arthritis. This year, thanks to Bikram, he became the U.S. men's yoga champion. Then there was Alisa Matthews, the reigning international women's champion, who'd been roped into competing by Bikram and Rajashree in 2004 because she was from Washington, D.C., and they'd needed a representative from there. Now she was finishing up a year of traveling around the world as an international yoga "ambassador," kind of like a yoga Miss America.

Just before the awarding of the international prizes, I met Courtney Mace, age thirty-two, from New York City. The previous day, she'd been crowned the U.S. women's champion, and today had executed a near-flawless routine capped by a magnificent crane pose. "The competition gets a lot of flak from a lot of people," she said, "but it's not like anyone's trying to crack anyone else's kneecaps. You're sharing your devotion, your story. Trying to help one another out."

A half-hour later, a bunch of buff dudes did a crass on-stage display of sweat-free yoga shorts invented by a Bikram studio owner. It looked like the Bikram series performed by Chippendale's dancers. Following that, Rajashree and Bikram awarded this year's prizes. The male title went to a sweet-looking gentleman from Singapore. Courtney Mace won the overall women's championship and would soon begin her travels as an international yoga ambassador.

The next morning, I went back to Mara's apartment, where I'd begun practicing again after a couple months off. The recession had been hard on hOM Yoga. Classes were smaller, and the modest accoutrements had grown even more bare-boned. On the floor above, Mara's neighbor appeared to be continually moving furniture, not to mention opening the screen door to his blue-plastic-tarp-covered patio several times an hour. No one else seemed to mind, but I found it hard to detach myself from the fact that I was practicing directly below an obsessive-compulsive lunatic.

Mara's cat rubbed against my chest while I was trying to do a headstand. If I practiced too close to her kitchen, sometimes I could smell the garbage. It was annoying.

At the same time, I was getting together with a small and trusted group of friends. There was no hero worship. We didn't compete, or talk about transformation or say that we wanted to teach yoga to the children; just some postures, some very light chanting, and a few laughs afterward. Sometimes we even went out for coffee after class.

I was damn glad to be there.

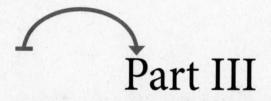

Part III

The Wind Blowing Around Inside of an Idiot

11

Pack Your Bag, I Don't Need the Ag

Because I was now a *Yoga Journal* contributor, it wasn't hard for me to get into the San Francisco *Yoga Journal* conference. As the magazine's PR person said, I had an "actual assignment." This made me wonder if people pretend to be journalists so they can sneak into yoga conferences. Was I just a fat, horny dude with a Spandex-and-chanting fetish, plus a press pass, or was I an actual bylined seeker of yogic truth? Did it matter? Regardless, I registered.

Yoga Journal sponsored its first-ever conference in Estes Park, Colorado, in 1996, and debuted at the Hyatt in downtown San Francisco in 2004. It now holds four conferences a year around the United States, with the Colorado and San Francisco ones constant and the other ones moving around to various locations such as New York, Boston, Florida, and Lake Geneva, Wisconsin (summer home to thousands of Chicago boat owners with mob connections). The conferences feature workshops from prominent teachers, lectures, many interesting demonstrations and entertainments, and a vast "yoga marketplace," altogether comprising a grand bazaar of enlightenment, new age bullshit, and everything in between. The conferences are also directly target-marketed at a tasty demographic that leans 85 percent female with a median age of thirty-six to forty-five and a median income of $80,000 a year, otherwise formerly known as the *Sex and the City* fan base.

I had several goals in attending the conference: I wanted to take the exact temperature of contemporary American yoga culture, and I wanted to improve my own yoga practice and knowledge. Perhaps most important, I wanted to get through the entire weekend for less than $200. Ordinarily, this wouldn't be possible. For the average attendee, the full four-day conference cost $965, or $820 if you did the early-bird registration. Hotel rooms at the Hyatt cost at least $211 a night. Then you had to consider airfare and food, and suddenly you were staring down a weekend yoga holiday for two grand. Most of the yoga people I knew couldn't afford that.

I'd already scored the free ticket. I'd been to San Francisco often enough to know how to do food on the cheap. And my lodging was secured when my *Yoga Journal* editor agreed to let me stay with her and her boyfriend.

"Why are you always such good friends with your editors?" Regina asked.

"Because I'm a thoroughgoing professional," I said.

"It's mostly the women editors you're friends with, not so much the men."

"Well," I said, slapping her on the ass, "I love the ladies, and the ladies love me."

"Fuck off, Pollack," she said.

Transportation was the final piece to my cheapness puzzle. Sure, I could fly into Oakland out of Burbank for something like $120 round-trip, but that still qualified as money. If I drove, on the other hand, I could get there and back on three tanks of gas. If I had carpool mates, I wouldn't have to pay anything at all. So I went to the conference website, which had a bulletin board for hotel room and ride shares. Someone named "Amy/Sat Prem" was looking for a ride up from L.A. From the "Sat" in front of her yoga name, I guessed that she fell into the *kundalini* camp. We started exchanging emails.

"Are you providing the car, and I'm paying gas?" she wrote. "I have an old Volvo, not sure it would be as comfortable as your transportation . . ."

Nearly erect at the prospect of not having to pay for gas, I wrote her back within fifteen seconds. Perhaps I overshared. The email went:

Well, I do have a Prius, but my wife is probably gonna want it while I'm gone. My other option is a 1998 Nissan Sentra. It gets decent mileage, but only has cassette. Don't know if that trumps the Volvo or not. Obviously, if I get the Prius, then I'm behind the wheel.

I'm staying with a friend and we can probably figure out a way to park the car near her place. Do you
want to nail this down and then look for a third carpool
friend over the next few weeks? Might as well turn it
into a party.

From your moniker, I take it you're a *kundalini* practitioner. I'm a *hatha/ashtanga* guy myself, but am interested in everything.

Namaste,

Neal

Sat Prem didn't respond. I began to worry that I'd
played my hand poorly. Had I erred in mentioning the fact
that the Nissan only had a cassette player? Maybe she was
a music snob. Then I realized that my suggestion to "turn it
into a party" might have come across like some sort of in-
vitation for weird yoga swinging. Or perhaps I just sounded
like I was afraid of my wife. Of course, it was none of those
things. She wrote me back weeks later and said that she'd
been in Costa Rica for the month of December and was just
now going through emails. Also, she'd decided to fly.

By then, though, it didn't matter, because I'd found my
carpool.

I put up my own post on the bulletin board, taking
great care to make myself sound as normal and neutral as
possible:

> *Looking for a carpool partner or two for the confer-
> ence. Can leave Thursday and would prefer to come
> back Sunday night or maybe Monday. Inquire above.*
>
> *Cheers!*

It took five days, but I got a response from someone named "Dhyana," though I don't know why I'm putting that in quotes because it's her actual name. She said she'd be "up for sharing costs," but it would only be one-way because she was staying in San Francisco after the conference. I wrote back, "Sounds like a plan. I don't know which car I'm using . . . neither is a guzzler, but the Prius is a nicer ride overall than my mother's old Nissan Sentra. What part of town do you call home?" Clearly, I had some insecurity issues when it came to the Nissan, an unspectacular but perfectly serviceable second car.

She wrote back, "I call home St. Norbert, Winnipeg, Canada. So it may be a little far for you to pick me up." However, she said, while in L.A. she'd be staying in Hollywood, near the Golden Bridge Yoga Center. That was reasonably close to my house, and right down the street from where my kid went to school. I wrote back, "it will be inexpensive, we will both bring healthy snacks and a reusable water container, and we're good! My only stipulation is: No *kirtan* on the way up! I'm a *hatha* guy." *Kirtan* is devotional yoga singing, and despite my devotion to the practice, I hadn't developed a taste.

"No worries about the *kirtan*," she wrote back. " I can wean myself off . . . the only *bhakti* praise I'll be singing is "thank the Lord it's not –40 degrees Celsius."

My life had degenerated to the point where I was now exchanging cornball yoga-and-weather quips with a stranger over email. Then the conversation moved over to Facebook, where we became friends. Two days after Christmas, Dhyana wrote, "A friend of mine might want to carpool, a fellow yogini and wild woman." This friend was named Denise, who Dhyana later described as "a fun character, die-hard yogini, and thrill seeker. Great heart. We're both pretty low key."

Well, that sounded like fun!

Soon after that, Denise also became my Facebook friend. They'd be staying in Hollywood with a couple of Canadian fashion designers named Chip and Pepper. I'd pick them up the morning we left.

Because of all the *kundalini* references in the emails and Facebook messages, I imagined my carpool mates as turbaned vegan asetics. A lot of Sikhs practice *kundalini,* so at parties, I started throwing around phrases like, "I'm carpooling up to San Francisco with a couple of Sikhs from Winnipeg. Isn't that wild?" Then I looked at Dhyana and Denise's pages on Facebook. They weren't, in fact, Sikhs at all.

"So," I said to Regina at dinner the night before the conference, "these women I'm driving to San Francisco . . ."

"I thought you were driving up with a couple of Indian guys."

"You don't have to be Indian to be Sikh," I said. "Also, they're not Sihks. They're Canadian."

"So, let me get this straight," she said. "You're driving two Canadian women to San Francisco by yourself?"

"Yep."

A vast silence ensued, during which Regina weighed the possibilities of divorce.

"*30 Rock* was really funny last night, huh?" I said.

The silence continued.

That night, I received an email from Dhyana. Chip and Pepper hadn't quite panned out. Instead, she said, they were going to stay at a cheap motel somewhere in Hollywood. As soon as I read that phrase, I knew what had to be done. I went upstairs to talk to Regina.

"Babe," I said. "These Canadian gals are going to stay at a motel in Hollywood, and I just don't think they should."

Regina sighed the deep, exasperated, permanent sigh of someone who knows that they've made a lifelong commitment to living with a massive pain in the ass.

"Fine," she said. "How many nights?"

"Just one," I said.

"I know it's the right thing to do," she said. "Still . . ."

"They're yoga people," I said. "They won't steal anything."

"I'm hiding my jewelry just in case," she said.

"Whatever you want, dear," I said, pausing briefly to let her think she was being accommodated before adding, "By the way, I'm taking the Prius."

We had pretty makeshift guest accommodations. One of the gals would sleep on Elijah's bottom bunk, and the other would shack up on the living room couch. They arrived just before dinnertime, and we had steaming plates of risotto waiting for them. It had been a long travel day, full of inevitable January Canadian weather delays, and they seemed grateful.

"Wow," Denise said. "The airport van kept driving, and the neighborhoods just kept getting posher and posher."

We lived one block away from a major high school and shared a driveway with our next-door neighbor. Also, we had no central air and our lone bathroom hadn't been redecorated since the protagonists of *Grey Gardens* were young. I didn't exactly consider our setup posh. But I guess compared to where they would have stayed otherwise, this was Shutters on the Beach.

Over dinner, we learned about our guests. Dhyana, who seemed very calm, lived communally at an art center in suburban Winnipeg, where she worked as the yoga teacher. She'd done a two-hundred-hour teacher training at a Sivananda center in the Bahamas, but she was always trying to improve her practice and knowledge. To that end, she'd obtained scholarships for three separate meditation retreats in Northern California that would occur after the conference, and she'd be traveling for a month. Her provincial government had given her a "young entrepreneur" grant to attend, as part of a program to try to keep young professionals in Manitoba. *Yeah, good luck with that,* I thought, while also thinking, *really, the Canadian government gave you a grant to study yoga?* Her suitcase contained mostly vitamins, plus a yoga block.

Denise resided in the mountains of Alberta, where she spent much of her time skiing. A great fan of the Zeitgeist series of conspiracy documentaries, she seemed continually to need to regulate with cigarettes, coffee, and gum, which she consumed in quick bursts of nervous energy. She'd done some hard living. As for the conference, she'd paid something like sixty bucks to attend two classes and one lecture, and planned to spend the rest of the time hitting the free stuff. She wasn't entirely sure how she was getting home, and didn't seem too concerned.

"So why did you come?" I said.

"Because I'm a fan of that song . . ." and she sang, "If you're going to San Franciscooooo . . . be sure to wear lots of flowers in your hair."

"Yeah, but that was 1967," I said, "and even then it was a cliché. San Francisco's not like that anymore."

"I'm looking forward to hanging with my homies in the Haight," she said.

"The Haight is mostly full of frat boys," I said.

But she didn't seem to believe me. She was naïve about the ways of California, though I'm sure that I'd be equally naïve about the ways of Western Canada were I to visit there on a whim. Regardless, I realized that of the three people in my carpool to the yoga conference, one was attending on a government grant, one had scored a press freebie, and the third had decided to attend without paying at all. I took pride in our collective cheapness.

After dinner, we went to Trader Joe's for road-trip supplies. I knew exactly what I wanted: beef jerky, chocolate, popcorn, seltzer, and sour Jelly Bellies. Dhyana strolled dreamily down the vitamin aisle, in search of a particular health supplement. Denise darted through the aisles like a computer-guided torpedo, but she didn't put anything in her basket. I waited by the checkout line for a while. Finally, Dhyana appeared with her vitamins and some yogurt.

"You're going to bring yogurt in my car?" I said.

"Is that OK?" she said.

"But yogurt smells like *ass*," I said.

"Oh, come on," she said. "Who doesn't like yogurt?"

"I don't like anything white and creamy."

"That's weird."

"I didn't say it wasn't weird."

Denise appeared. Her basket was still empty.

"Oooh," she said. "Yogurt. Where'd you get that?"

"In the yogurt aisle," said Dhyana.

"That you walked by like thirty times," I said.

"I'll be right back," she said. Before I could look down, it seemed, she was back with her own yogurt. She was like the ADHD Flash.

"Are those jelly beans?" she asked.

"Yep," I said.

"No refined sugar for me, thanks. It's really bad for you."

"It's my funeral," I replied.

"True enough," she said. "Oooooh! Did you get chocolate?"

"Yes."

"I want some!"

"You can have some."

"Do they have fruit here?"

"It's right behind you," I said.

I rolled my eyes. Dhyana rolled her eyes. Denise rolled her eyes. Already, we were on one another like siblings. When we finally left the store, Denise looked around twitchily.

"How long will it take to walk to your house from here?" she said. Good lord. She was like a restless Doberman puppy.

"Fifteen, twenty minutes," I said.

"That's exactly the amount of walking I need," she said.

I gave her the best directions I could.

"You want to come?" she said to Dhyana.

Dhyana regarded her sleepily.

"No thanks," she said. "I've been traveling for twenty-one straight hours."

About forty-five minutes later, Denise showed up at my

front door. She'd gotten a little lost on the way over. Also, she'd met some very interesting people on the street.

"I told them I was *going to San Franciscoooooo. . . . and I was going to wear flowers in my hair,*" she sang.

"That's enough with the singing," I said.

She unrolled her yoga mat in my living room and began doing all kinds of crazy stretches.

"My chakras are totally fucking out of whack," she said.

It was time for bed. Lying there, Regina implored me to be careful driving the next day. No fiddling with the iPod while the car was moving, she said.

"So you're gonna get in around noon or one?" she asked.

"No, more like early evening."

"It doesn't take twelve hours to drive to San Francisco."

"It does if you take the Pacific Coast Highway."

"Dude, you are *not* taking Highway 1 all the way up. That road is dangerous."

"But it's beautiful. Come on. I-5 is totally *not* yoga."

"Fuck yoga," she said.

"So it's come to that," I said.

"You're going to do what you want, aren't you?"

"I'll be fine," I said.

"You always say you'll be fine."

"And I'm always fine."

"Until you're not."

She sighed.

"Fine, go drive up Highway 1 with your girlfriends to your yoga conference. I'll just stay here and take care of our son."

"Don't make me feel guilty."

"I'm not making you feel anything."

"Yes you are."

"I'm a yoga widow."

But really, I'd only be gone for three days. Plus, it wasn't costing us anything, and like the lady at *Yoga Journal* said, I had an "actual assignment." Also, if my interactions with the ladies thus far were any indication, it's not like my road trip was going to be a continuation of the last scene of *Dazed and Confused*.

Everyone was up by 7 AM. I went into the living room. Denise had been doing her stretches for an hour and now she really needed a smoke. Dhyana sat at our dining-room table, placidly drinking a cup of coffee. Elijah sat next to her, turning a liquid hourglass thing back and forth, like a college kid tripping in his dorm room.

"Elijah," Dhyana said. "We have something for you."

She reached into her backpack and pulled out a Dream catcher.

"It's what Native Canadians use to capture their dreams," she said. "Pretty cool, right?"

He regarded it for a minute.

"I'm going to put this in my room, right now!" he said.

He dashed away. Weren't they sweet to get him a present? Regina emerged last, in her bathrobe. I'd already loaded the car, taking care to put the yogurt in tightly sealed smell-proof containers. Reg gave me a gentle kiss on the lips.

"Yoga on, dude," she said. "Be careful."

"OK," I said.

"And have fun."

"Thanks, babe."

And thus, with the blessing of my kind, loving, and patient wife, I drove off into the rising dawn with my

Canadian carpool mates, ready for whatever the day might bring.

Two hours into the drive, we decided to stop at a beach. It was a glorious January morning and Midwestern Canada wouldn't see anything like this until mid-July. It was the diametric opposite of the frozen wastelands of Manitoba. This was my special treat to the ladies. We could have chosen many beaches along the way, but I had one in mind: Refugio State Beach, just north of Santa Barbara. I'd always liked Refugio because it felt authentically seashorey, even though it was fronted by a sizable and popular RV camp-ground. It had palm trees at sand's edge and a nifty set of tide pools on the northern tip. The beach-keepers kept it in a natural state, which meant no sand grooming or shell-and-seaweed removal.

We arrived at the guard gate.

"That's nine dollars," said the ranger.

"NINE DOLLARS!" Denise said.

Dhyana relaxedly reached for her wallet. I could see the mild discomfort on her face. Clearly, we comprised a cheap-assed road crew. But we should pay, I said to them; it's worth the money.

"Beaches should be free," said Denise.

Freaking Canadians, always looking for a handout. They already got government-funded health care and grants to study yoga. What else did they want? But the second I parked, no one complained about money anymore. The Ca-nadian ladies gleefully galloped toward the water like pup-pies taken off-leash at the dog run.

While they gamboled merrily, I squirreled into my

bathing suit in the backseat. When I emerged, Dhyana was sitting placidly on her heels in the sand, palms up, and, with her eyes closed, had beatifically turned her face up toward the sun. I couldn't tell which was shining brighter, her face or the sun. How, I wondered, could anyone appear so peaceful, even on a quiet morning like this? Meanwhile, a way down the beach, Denise stood with her legs apart, swinging her arms wildly across her body, making huffing noises. This, apparently, was how she relaxed. She was virtually exploding with energy, as though my car had been a prison.

Well, I couldn't let my guests do yoga on the beach without showing off my *own* chops. I moved backward onto the grass, and my arms swooped upward into a sun salutation. I went through the whole A series several times, dropping down, bending forward, lifting up, and rising again, while Dhyana meditated and Denise did her ape-woman routine.

Eventually, Dhyana snapped out of it, but Denise kept going. We approached her warily. I asked,

"What are you doing?"

"It's the Breath of Joy, man!" she said.

This was new to me, I told her.

"You gotta do the Breath of Joy!" she said.

She showed me: You swoop your arms back, and then when you swing them forward, you expel your breath, almost violently, or at least with a grunt. Meanwhile, sway those hips. Make it forceful. Breathe like you mean business.

That's how the three of us came to stand on that beach in Santa Barbara stomping and huffing like a bunch of tourists performing some sort of native Maori dance celebration. It was a new low point, or possibly high point, in my yoga life. Here I was, doing silly things in public without judging myself, without suffocating cynicism, without air quotes around everything. The Breath of Joy probably wasn't something I'd go back to regularly. I still had boundaries, for fuck's sake! But for that moment, at that time, with that glorious sun glowing on my face, it would do just fine. It had been more than twenty years since I'd felt this way. This was the kind of thing we'd done back at good old Anytown, USA; this was the moment in *City Slickers* where Billy Crystal, annoyingly, found his smile.

"That's it! That's it!" Denise said. "Work it out! Do the Breath of Joy!"

This was my reality now. I belonged here.

Afterward, in the car, I attempted to explain my yoga journey to my newfound yoga mates.

"Well, um, one of the things about yoga, you know, the term *namaste,* how it means my best self honors your best self and all, well, I wasn't really my best self a few years ago because I started this rock band and then I had a kid and there was, like, this total identity shift, and then the *New York Times* called me fat and I kind of had this nervous breakdown. So my wife got me into yoga and I did it a little bit at a time until we moved to Los Angeles and then one day I was opening my birthday presents and . . ."

In the back, Denise had fallen asleep. Dhyana listened patiently. I continued:

"So then I was like, you know what, I've been my best self before, in high school and occasionally other times, and I'm going to go searching for that best version of myself, through yoga. Does that make sense?"

"Sort of," Dhyana said.

"It's a pretty sincere quest, even though I have no idea what I'm looking for."

"Well," she said, "at least you're honest."

About thirty miles down the road, we stopped at another beach to watch the elephant seals. It was high mating season. You haven't lived until you've watched an elephant-seal beach orgy. The male seals, with their bulbous, spreading noses, mounted the females violently, making a low, guttural, horrifically desperate noise that sounded like nighttime in the apnea ward of a sleep-disorders clinic. What this had to do with yoga, I don't know, but I do know that it represented our last peaceful road-trip moment before the bickering started.

We stopped in a town for food. The ladies wanted to avoid wheat. Dhyana refused sugar because it was "an evil industry."

"Totally," I said, shoving a handful of sour Jelly Bellies in my mouth.

We drove past a couple of options but they rejected each one, until Denise emerged from a gas station brandishing a bran muffin. It didn't go over well in the car. We each ate about two bites before the muffin went into the discard pile with our other half-consumed snacks. At this point, the road got narrow and unpopulated. There'd be no food for hours.

Denise grabbed the iPod from the front seat. She whooped.

"WHOOOOOO!" she said. "You've *12 Golden Country Greats*! Turn it up, dude!"

She was referring to the classic Ween album comprised of country songs that aren't exactly country songs. To show that she had good taste, she turned to the best of the best, *Piss up a Rope*. This song, which contains the lyrics "you can wash my balls with a warm wet rag" and "I'm sick of your mouth and your two-percent milk," is about the rudest, most sexist, and most awesome country-music parody ever written. Denise and I realized it, and paid appropriate trib-ute. As we curved along Highway 1, we sang, "Pack your bag, I don't need the ag, on your knees you big booty bitch start suckin' . . ."

"Oh my!" Dhyana exclaimed. "Those aren't yoga lyrics!"

We drove on. There were rockslide delays. Sometimes, a view took away my breath and we just had to stop. Every time, Denise ran around the parking lot like we'd been keeping her in a five-point harness. Finally, we arrived at Big Sur, the most beautiful place of all. We saw the first restaurants we'd encountered in hours. Denise told us to drive on.

"I want to get to *San Franciscooooooooo* . . ." she sang.

"What I don't think you understand," I said, "is that while San Francisco is a great city, you're going to probably spend tonight wandering around a shitty tourist neighbor-hood with a bunch of shitty tourists. On the other hand, this is the most beautiful drive in the world, and I don't think you're appreciating it." *Young lady.*

"*I'm going to wear lots of flowers in my hair. . . .*"

"Seriously, dude, don't sing that fucking song again!"

"I will sing whatever I want to sing!"

Dhyana ran her hands over her face. We all felt very hungry. *Dharma Bums*, this wasn't.

Over the next six hours, I: pulled into the Esalen Insti-tute only to be informed that their legendary waters were only open to the public at 3 AM, and even then you had to be very quiet; drove to an outlet mall north of Monterey at Denise's insistence because she wanted to get a sandwich from the deli of a discount grocery store; listened to three increasingly worried voice-mail messages from Regina, received when out of range; turned onto the 101 because Denise was basically screaming at me that she wanted to *get to San Francisco now*; stopped at the entrance to an RV Park so Denise could urinate in the bushes; ate at a strip-mall Panera Bread, where Dhyana took a very long time assessing the nutritional content of everything before she ordered, then tried to pay with Canadian dollar coins; got a wicked back massage from Denise in the Panera parking lot, as, after 11 hours of driving, I was clearly showing signs of wear; tried to placate Regina on the phone while in harrowing Berkeley-area traffic; got a neck rub from Dhyana in the backseat when certain muscles began to visibly spasm; tried to understand a bunch of jokes about ayurvedic healing; dropped the ladies off at their sketchy-looking hotel on the border of Union Square and the Tenderloin; thought, *holy God, after today I'm going to need a shitload of yoga.*

My wishes were soon fulfilled.

A shitload of yoga is exactly what I got.

Karma, Aligned

I staggered through the chilly, misty streets of the Financial District sometime not too long after dawn. My yoga mat was slung over my right shoulder, a patterned wool blanket, borrowed from my teacher, was wedged between the strap and my side. Over my other shoulder I carried a tattered messenger bag that had been quite stylish during the first dot-com boom. It contained a towel, a notebook, a yoga strap, a tennis ball, and a little beef jerky in case I got peckish during a session. Since getting to San Francisco, I'd lost feeling in the tip of my left thumb. My lower back ached, my forehead leaked sweat, and my throat was dry and scratchy. I felt shaggy and diseased. Driving for twelve hours the day before had clearly ruined my body. I was like a new-age mule, beaten and bowed.

Down Market Street, I could see the Hyatt Regency, a gray, prison-like structure with narrow slitted windows, the type of building that had gone up in the late '60s and early '70s to keep out the hippies. Now, of course, hippies overran the place, except that the hippies were old, and they had money to burn. From every street, at every angle, they walked toward the hotel-fortress, gliding with serenity and confidence. I fell in next to one of them. She was visiting from Idaho, where she lived a life of peace and rustic luxury.

"You going to the conference?" I asked.

"Oh, yes, I go every year," she said. "I've been doing yoga since the '60s. I used to practice with a two-dimensional poster. I got all the poses wrong. But I hung in there until the videos came along."

Lurching through the doors of the Hyatt, I entered a sea of crazy old ladies seeking their next *kundalini* high, as well as a decent number of smokin' hot babes in tight lululemon pants. A few men floated about carefully, like Triassic-era furry mammals looking for eggs to gnaw, not wanting to disturb the dominant species. Everyone seemed excited and awake. I was a midnight guy in the Valley of the Morning People. My conference would begin with an all-day "intensive" called The Yogi As Radical Cultural Hero, taught by David Life and Sharon Gannon, the founders of Jivamukti Yoga in New York. Now, this may seem like a strange choice, given that my previous experience at Jivamukti ended with me storming, in a drug-filled rage, into the Union Square dusk. The conference offered at least a half-dozen other all-day workshops that probably would have suited me better. But I had my reasons for choosing this one.

For one thing, I felt guilty, as though I'd done something wrong by not giving the Jivamukti method a chance, particularly since I'd gone in completely ignorant. Since then, I'd done a little reading. Jivamukti still didn't seem like my style, but at least I'd have the opportunity to reject it with knowledge. Second, I've always considered myself a bit of a cultural hero, but had recently slipped on the heroism front and was looking for fresh pointers. Third, I *was* writing a book about yoga culture. Skipping a workshop called The Yogi As Radical Cultural Hero in favor of an eight-hour class on back-care basics would probably have been better for my overall physical and mental health, but it wouldn't do much service to the narrative. So I picked the juicy low-lying fruit.

My yoga intensive took place in a medium-sized conference room partitioned by sliding walls in the Hyatt's sub-basement. Someone had gotten up very early that morning to carefully apply blue masking tape to the carpet, creating neat, evenly measured rows of rectangular spaces each large enough for a yoga mat and some miscellaneous props. The room had low, cheap-looking ceiling tiles and ample fluorescent overhead lighting. Was I about to do yoga, or listen to a bunch of boring speeches from drug-company sales reps?

I chose my rectangle, middle-back, on the right side. Too close up, I might have appeared like a kiss-ass, and too far back, I might have seemed disinterested. This, to me, made for a suitably skeptical distance. My top layers came off, and there I sat under the conference-room lights, in my yoga shorts and tank top, ready to absorb wisdom.

David Life and Sharon Gannon, eyes serenely closed, hands in *anjali mudra,* meditated on pillows at the front of the room. He was ribs-showing thin, with sallow cheekbones, a ponytail, and black disk earrings, kind of like the yoga version of Iggy Pop. She just looked happy, healthy, and attractive. For lack of a better celebrity comparison, let's say Anjelica Huston.

As people trickled into the room, the gurus stood. With simple, kind grins, they moved from person to person with their palms together at their chests, bowing like Japanese businesspeople in a boardroom. Only about thirty of us had arrived by that point, but they bowed at least a dozen times. Several young female assistants accompanied Life and Gannon in their bowing. Hotness shone through their weird gestures. In fact, they were so adorable that I considered going into the hall and dumping a cup of ice water down my pants so I could properly focus.

When that all was over, the assistants passed out two fliers. One was a press release for Gannon's new book *Yoga and Vegetarianism: The Diet of Enlightenment*, with her and Life's traveling teacher schedule on the back. The other contained ads for more Jivamukti books, as well as a list of 2009's Jivamukti Yoga Chants.

Then Life ordered us to the wall and told us to hold handstand for twenty breaths. I hadn't yet reached the point in my practice where this was possible, but I tried. Physical activation is spiritual activation, he told us. There should be a little discomfort, because in the face of discomfort we transform ourselves, just like Martin Luther King Jr. had done. I think I got his point, though I doubted that Dr. King thought up the Montgomery Bus Boycott while *schvitzing* all over himself during repeated attempts to flip into handstand.

We went back to our mats and sat in *virasana,* or hero pose.

"A hero's quest is to retrieve something that has been lost," Life said.

Like my best self, I thought.

"You have the power in your voice to alter your physical surroundings," he continued. "That's why all great heroes were also great public speakers. They started talking great uplifting words and didn't waste their time complaining."

Well, now I just felt guilty. I spent 80 percent of my life complaining. Maybe these people were onto something. I thought about this as I sat cross-legged in the basement of the Hyatt Regency San Francisco, chanting *shanti shanti shanti* over and over again.

Now Gannon sat down at her harmonium and took control of the room. "We have to see ourselves as cultural heroes," she said, "dramatic entities. We have to transform ourselves from ordinary people to Supermen and women. We have to work magic in order to enact transformation."

Oh, good grief, I thought. *Here we go.*

"Yoga is that state where you're not missing anything," she said. "You are whole and complete."

She asked us to refer to our chant sheet, began playing her harmonium, and sang:

Lokah Samastah Sukhino Bavantu

This was familiar to me. Mara sometimes chanted this

at the end of our Ashtanga classes. Along with everyone else, I chanted back:

Lokah Samastah Sukhino Bavantu

Underneath that chant, in bold letters, were some words in English. I figured those were just there for translation purposes, but no. She chanted, in the same voice and rhythm:

May all beings everywhere be happy and free and may the thoughts, words, and actions of my own life contribute in some way to that happiness and to that freedom for all.

Now, this was a fine sentiment. But chanting it call-and-response felt one step away from putting on the purple sneakers and asking the aliens to come and get me. In general, English, a fine language for profanity, political speeches, and broadcasting baseball games, is a poor translation choice for profound lyrical sentiments from ancient texts. To wit: the subtle humiliations of *shul,* which I attend in the reform tradition because the services are pretty short. When I chant Hebrew prayers, I feel like I'm tapping into an ancient culture of devotion, bonded through ritual to multiple generations of long-forgotten ancestors. When I try the prayers in English, it sounds like I'm reading promotional copy for Yahweh, Inc. The same applies to Sanskrit, which says beautifully, in three or four words, that which requires seemingly endless blather in my native tongue.

So when Gannon chanted *Sthira suhham asanam,* I chanted back. But when she chanted *the connection to the earth should be steady and joyful. Our relationships with all beings and things should be mutually beneficial if we ourselves desire happiness and liberation from suffering. No true or lasting happiness can come from causing unhappiness to others,* my mind wandered. No one else in the room seemed to care, though. The canvas-and-plastic walls vibrated with their joined voices, while I sat on my mat, silently complaining.

The rest of the morning went as follows: Vigorous, sweaty *vinyasa;* lecture about the ethics of vegetarianism; and profound chat about what it means to be a hero. While standing on my head, I heard things like "there's no more powerful force than your own perception of yourself. That will determine who you are." Gannon said, "don't think about the future or the past, just the present. You need to see people on your equal level. See the happiness of the other that you're speaking to so that they become happy in your presence. That's love, divinity. The possibilities are limitless."

Around this point, I realized that one of Life's and Gannon's hot assistants looked familiar. Could it be? *Oh, yes,* I thought, *it could.* She was my archenemy from New York, the teacher with whom I'd argued on my worst yoga day ever. Suddenly, my decision to take The Yogi As Radical Cultural Hero had a true purpose.

I could redeem one of the most irredeemable encounters in my life. What an opportunity! *I would make her happy in my presence.* It wasn't exactly Martin Luther King Jr.–worthy. Hell, it wasn't even Harry Reid–worthy. But it still felt like the right thing to do.

When they announced lunch break, I went up to my yoga nemesis.

"Um, hi," I said.

"Hi," she said.

"So yeah, I just wanted to say, well, um, I took your class at Jivamukti one time and, like, um, the politics sort of freaked me out, and I totally stormed out of the room. I had a huge temper tantrum and was just so pissed off. Also, I was on drugs. You probably don't remember."

"I *totally* don't remember," she said.

"Well, I just want to apologize."

"No need to apologize," she said. "You're still here, aren't you?"

"I guess I am."

"There's no tension now, is there?"

"I guess not."

She opened her arms for a big hug. I gladly accepted her embrace.

Mmm, I thought. *You smell nice.*

"There we go," I said.

She passed a hand, palm down, in front of her waist.

"Karma . . . aligned." she said.

Now I was a radical cultural hero.

An hour and a half later, I returned to the conference, my belly full of pork. This felt a little blasphemous, but all that yoga and talk of vegetarian ethics made me very hungry. It could have been worse; my appetite had craved a steak or double burger. I showed great restraint in only ordering a BLT with deliciously marbled Niman Ranch bacon.

We took our seats.

"Did anyone do anything kind over lunch?" Life asked.

I nodded my head nonchalantly. Teacher called on me. *Wait*, I thought. *I didn't mean to participate.*

"What did you do?" he asked.

"I gave someone some of my ice cream."

"Sharing food," he said, obviously disappointed with my third-grade answer.

But it was true. I'd ordered a big honking bowl of sorbetto at the Ferry Building, and had given some to a random person at the conference. I didn't tell Life this, though. Instead, I said,

"It was non-dairy ice cream."

Don't tell him you ate bacon, I thought.

The second half of our intensive featured a special guest.

"He's hot!" Gannon said. "He's hip! He's holy! Please put your hands together for MC Yogi G!"

A white guy strolled to the center of the room. His hair and beard were buzzed close. His mustard-yellow T-shirt bore the image of a Native American who had the Stars and Stripes drawn over his mouth. He had a calm smile and sleepy, knowing eyes.

"What up, yoga people," he said.

MC Yogi, the yoga trend of the moment, had arrived.

The creation myth of MC Yogi goes as follows: Nicolas Giacomini spent most of his teenage years living in a group-home for at-risk youth in Northern California. He made it through by writing his own raps and performing them for his friends at house parties. At age eighteen, his father invited him to practice yoga with a group of friends in a converted storeroom behind a place called Toby's Feed Barn. There he began a lifelong study of the yogic arts, culminating with a teacher training in 2000, where he met his impossibly beautiful wife. They traveled to India together and returned home to open a yoga studio in Point Reyes.

With some variation, you hear the same story about the founding of just about every neighborhood yoga studio in the world. However, this one diverged when young Nicolas began putting his yoga knowledge into rhyme to create, according to his website, "an exciting new sound that brings the wisdom of yoga to a whole new generation of modern mystics and urban yogis." On September 9, 2008, he released his first full-length album, *Elephant Power,* and its breakout single, "Ganesh Is Fresh." Suddenly an ordinary neighborhood yoga teacher found himself in demand at yoga conferences around the world. He was yoga's Eminem. A global tour schedule began to develop, and a full-on yoga career was born.

Of course, when it comes to yoga music, even the highest-level performer draws about as well as a mid-level indie rock band's side project, and so MC Yogi found himself, at two on a Friday afternoon, performing in front of thirty people in the basement of the Hyatt Regency.

MC Yogi began by reciting his song "Be the Change," about the ultimate radical cultural hero, the Mahatma himself. When it came time for the chorus, the whole class sang along:

"Be the change that you wanna see in the world, just like Gandhi!"

How the hell did they know the words? Were people really singing along to a rap about Gandhi? Could I go home now?

The song went on for quite a while, going into great specificity about Gandhi's life (*The biggest event that made the British halt/is when Gandhi G decided to harvest salt*) and encouraging us to follow our hearts to become great.

To MC Yogi's credit, he didn't try to rhyme anything with the word "Mahatma," the Hindi-English transliteration version of "orange."

When he was finished rapping, MC Yogi said, "there are two things that every radical cultural hero has in common: *sangha,* or community, and *sandra,* or practice." We had our community right here, he said. As he said that, I looked over at my former archenemy. She winked at me, which I thought was a little weird.

Now, said MC Yogi, it was time to practice. Since he was a certified yoga teacher, or, as he amusingly put it, "certifiable," he'd lead us in some *vinyasa* for a while.

"You should freestyle teach!" Gannon said. "Go MC Yogi!"

"What does that mean?" said MC Yogi.

"Freestyle rap while you teach."

MC Yogi decided this was a good idea. As he walked through the rows, he said, "*Drishdi* and *bandha* channeling the *prana*/from the base of the spine to the third-eye chakra." Fortunately or not, I understood exactly what he was talking about.

At one point, MC Yogi had us do a complicated balancing pose. The assistants walked around the room, helping. As I tried to balance, I started to tip backward, then forward, and then I totally collapsed. My former enemy caught me and put me straight.

"I saved you," she said.

"Don't let it go to your head," I said.

All good freestyle yoga rap *vinyasa* classes must come to an end, and MC Yogi eventually took a seat. We were winding up our day together, and Gannon said she wanted

everyone to draw together close in a circle, so we could process. Afterward, she said, there would be "ecstatic dancing."
My testicles began to shrivel.

Gannon called for questions.

A soft-spoken middle-aged man raised his hand.

"You write a lot about meat and dairy alternatives,"
he said, "but I've heard that too much soy is dangerous for
women's estrogen levels. Can you address that?"

All right, enough for me, then! I've always vowed to
never sit in a circle talking about estrogen levels, followed
by ecstatic dancing. Now I knew the truth: Life and Gannon
were excellent teachers who operated at the highest level,
but there'd be no more Jivamukti for me. Instead, I'd go
home and get stoned. The night's activities promised to be
huge.

Two weeks before the conference was supposed to start,
attendees got an email announcing that a Friday evening
class had been added to the schedule. It was called Move
and Be Moved: Music and Yoga with Michael Franti, Nicki
Doane, and Eddie Modestini. If you live in Northern
California or attend jam-band festivals, you'll be familiar with the dreadlocked, magnetically handsome Franti.
His band, Spearhead, travels the world mixing hip hop
with a variety of other styles, including funk, reggae, jazz,
folk, and rock, all while spinning out a politically conscious good-time vibe for his fan base. In recent years, he's
become the patron musical saint of yoga culture and the
most famous practitioner in the yoga-as-live-music scene.
A few weeks before the conference, I'd conducted a highly
intimate email interview with Franti for my *Yoga Journal*

story. "I really look at my performances as yoga—a way to connect heart mind and body with other hearts minds and bodies," he wrote.

When Franti goes on tour, he visits a different yoga studio in every city, which he says is "a really amazing way to the see the country." He's building the "Stay Human Yoga Retreat Center" in Bali (where he'll also have a recording studio), has started a yoga-inspired apparel company called "Stay Human" (whose clothes, he says, have "street edge" and "attitude"), and is looking to add a yoga component to the live-music festival, Power to the Peaceful, that he throws every September in Golden Gate Park.

Doane and Modestini, the other headliners in "Move and Be Moved," are a husband-and-wife teaching team, both certified by Patthabi Jois in Mysore before it was super-trendy. They live and teach in Maui and in Sebastopol, California, a setup that would inspire envy except that true yogis don't experience envy, so instead it's just awesome. They met Franti through a mutual friend when they went to see him at a music festival. Yoga followed, and there was an instant connection. Franti invited Doane and Modestini to his house in San Francisco. He visited them on Maui and played music during *savasana* for them.

Then they went on a three-week tour with Franti and Ziggy Marley, doing yoga on beer-soaked barroom floors, ratty green-room carpets, and in the parking lot by the tour bus. This came naturally to Doane, because she used to travel with the Dead. After that, whenever Doane and Modestini were on the road and happened to be in the same town as Franti, they'd hook up and yoga-and-music mania would ensue, always with fabulously moving results. But their show at the conference would be their biggest experiment yet.

I arrived a half-hour early. There were lines at every door to the Hyatt's main ballroom, which has a lot of doors. The entire hotel seemed to be overwhelmed by casually dressed people with yoga mats, jockeying for position. My pants were bunching into my ass. I smelled like bacon and weed. At times like this I remembered why I rarely left the house.

Finally, the doors opened. People poured into the grand ballroom from all directions. The entire hall had been partitioned with the conference's signature blue masking tape. This was exactly the way I hated to start a yoga class: in a mad rush for pole position. I took my usual skeptical spot in the middle, toward the back. Above me were bat mitzvah party lights in enormous beehive shapes. The carpet was luxuriously soft and dark-blue and probably got vacuumed sixteen times a day. Soon, every blue rectangle was filled. A couple of kids (whose parents were very busy taking pictures of each other), weaved between the mats, knocking over water bottles and grinning like they'd gotten away with eating rainbow-sprinkle-topped donuts for breakfast. I found myself getting very annoyed with my fellow conference attendees. Apparently, I wasn't the only one.

"Yoga isn't supposed to be entertaining," said a guy next to me.

"So why are you here, then?" I asked.

"Because I wanted to see Michael Franti," he said.

For some reason, I hadn't realized that a yoga class/concert featuring Michael Franti would have an audience largely comprised of his fans. I was, it seemed, the only person in the room unfamiliar with his oeuvre. Therefore, because I was vigorously doing *asana* instead of taking notes, I can't quote any of the song lyrics back to you, though I can tell you that the songs were mellow and kind during the easy opening warm-up poses. The music picked up speed and intensity alongside the practice, until, at one point I found myself in warrior one, clapping my hands overhead along with three hundred people who were singing along to a song about "rebel rockers."

Doane and Modestini roamed the crowd with their wireless microphones, leading us through tough poses that they made us hold for a very long time. She did most of the talking. This was obviously her party. Early on in the practice/concert, someone left the room on the far side. Doane blew her a kiss and said "I love you, sweetie." At another point, she said, "I love this! I love Michael, you all are here, all my friends are here. No one is getting more out of this than me."

Well, I certainly wasn't, but the rest of the crowd seemed to be enjoying itself. Cougar-age lululemon babes charged the stage during their favorite songs. There was much free-style grooving in the room. Then MC Yogi appeared on stage to perform his hit song from *Elephant Power*, "Ganesh Is Fresh."

As Franti played behind him, MC Yogi bounced around the stage pogo-style, with a happy yoga grin. When the chorus came along, he said, *when I say Jaya you say Ganesh!*

"Jaya!" he shouted

"Ganesh!" said the crowd.

"Jaya!"

"Ganesh!"

The musicians quickly switched gears to worshipping a more secular deity. Barack Obama's inauguration was only five days away. Franti had written a song to commemorate the rise of a new American day. He and MC Yogi performed it together. Everyone in the room threw up their hands as one and began to dance wildly as the chorus kicked in:

> *Barack Obama! Yes we can yeah!*
> *Barack Obama! We all come together now!*
> *Barack Obama! Ya ya ya! Barack Obama!*

This, I thought, *is exactly what the Republicans feared America would become*: an Eastern-tinged rave scene led by rich middle-aged liberals from San Francisco. The age of Obama and *Slumdog Millionaire* was upon us, a moment in time where limousine leftist politics, yoga, pop music, and casual name-dropping of Hindu deities had mixed into a cardamom incense-and-hope scented stew of self-righteous ecstasy. After eight years of the Bush presidency, this felt unsurprising, and maybe even a little necessary, but that didn't mean I was enjoying myself. I prefer my ecstatic states to occur in quieter, more private settings, where I can express a little snark and cynicism to show how uncomfortable they make me.

So even though my muscles were quivering for mercy when the *asana* ended, and even though Franti led us through a lovely *savasana,* I found myself not wanting to stick around for the encore. Plus, I was super-hungry and I really had to pee.

When I was done in the john, I went outside. I'd forgotten to tie the string to my yoga pants. As I reached my hand up to hail a cab, they fell down around my ankles. It appeared that, for me at least, the age of Obama would just be more of the same.

13

A Great Opportunity to Do Nothing

I tossed restlessly all night. My body felt like it was undergoing a continuous muscle spasm; I had more tics than a dog abandoned to the cruel streets of Cairo. At some point late in the night, my hosts came home noisily. They'd been celebrating a birthday at the Willie Nelson concert, and I found myself wishing that I'd been there.

Too soon came the dawn, and my 8 AM Saturday session. I'd registered for something called Finding Ease at Your Edge, but, once again, I sensed a disservice to the narrative: "And then I found ease at my edge," the end.

So instead I slipped in to something called The Sacred Geometry of Connection, run by the founders of AcroYoga, Jason Nemer and Jenny Sauer-Klein. AcroYoga, a discipline of growing popularity in California and beyond, combines exactly what the name implies. Nemer is a two-time U.S. junior acrobatic champion who performed in the Opening Ceremonies to the 1996 Olympic Games in Atlanta. Sauer-Klein comes from the contemporary "circus arts" movement, and is a great proponent of the physical art of yoga "flying."

This sounded possibly intriguing, and certainly vigorous. But when I got there, a little late, twenty people were sitting in a circle, holding hands. This was all part of AcroYoga, which begins each practice with a "Circle Ceremony," a time of contemplation and light hugging and coordinated hand movements. Says the AcroYoga website: "The circle initiates the ceremonious joining of our yoga community with a flow of integrated movements. Here we establish connection with those around us and cultivate our openness to the divine. The circle ceremony sets the tone and theme for our journey together."

It reminded me of the first fifteen minutes of the day in my son's first-grade classroom. The teacher calls roll, the kids each share something, they do a little light stretching. It's a great routine for first-graders. For me, though, the kind of yoga guy who would rather do anything than "partner work," not so much. The only things I like to share in yoga class are wisecracks and the smell of my unwashed mat. That's what I bring to the table.

Everyone was going around and sharing what was "sacred" to them. Most of the answers were what you might expect: nature, children, yoga, Barack Obama. The most interesting response came from a stocky older guy with thick glasses and a wild, nearly white beard. San Francisco is full of these late-Beat Era dudes who just keep going, alternative-culture Energizer bunnies. His name was Elliot, he said. He was a "transpersonal psychologist." Because of that, he said, "What is sacred to me is . . . well . . . evil!"

Now *that* I could get behind. But when the circle came to me, I deliberately faded into the wallpaper. Most things I found sacred, like marijuana, masturbating to Internet porn, and eating variety meats, simply weren't going to go over well during an 8 AM Saturday circle ceremony, and I certainly wasn't going to invoke the name of the Los Angeles Dodgers while in San Francisco. "I'm Neal," I said, "and my family is sacred to me."

Next, the circle leader invoked the Hindu Gods Sita and Ram. According to Hindu mythology, Ram is the seventh incarnation of the great Lord Vishnu, made manifest on Earth to free us from the cruelty and sins of the demon king Ravana. This was no small task, and, as a great hero, Ram needed love to get him through his trials. This came in the form of Sita, a hot little royal number who also happened to be the incarnation of Lakshmi, Lord Vishnu's "consort." Ram won Sita's hand in a contest during which he bent and broke Shiva's immortal bow. Many adventures followed, including some awesome battles led by the trickster monkey warrior god Hanuman, and after several hundred pages, Ram and Sita were joined on the throne of the world as great symbols of eternal love and compassion.

So, naturally, we had to chant their names at the Hyatt.

Sita, chanted the leader.

Sita, we chanted back.

Rama.

Rama.

Ohhhh Ram Ram Ram Sita Ram, Sita Ram.

Ohhhh Ram Ram Ram Sita Ram, Sita Ram.

This actually made me a little angry. I don't even believe in my *own* God, and here I was, being asked to blindly worship alternate deities like I was in some sort of Indian nursery school. In my notebook, I wrote, "I ain't no Hindu, man."

Next came a little *asana* to warm up the spine. We had to take partners. I was assigned to a handsome and fit fellow who, like me, was wearing a yoga tank top. One of us had to be Sita, the leader said, and one had to be Ram.

"What, is that like a top and bottom thing?" I said.

"You're Ram, and I'm Sita," my partner said huffily.

Now all ten pairs of Sitas and Rams needed to sit back to back. We were to lock elbows, sit up and lean back over each other. My partner instructed me every step of the way, because I, for some reason, couldn't understand what the teacher was saying.

"Have you done this before?" I asked him, as we undulated back and forth.

"I'm an AcroYoga teacher," he said.

I'd been *wondering* why he'd been nodding so enthusiastically whenever the leaders said anything. They called for a "triad," and asked for two AcroYoga teachers to help them. Half the room stepped forward. It was then that I realized I was out of my depth. The triad locked knees, joined hands, moved back and forth and up and down, flowing beautifully and rhythmically and semi-erotically, like the

cast of *All That Jazz* during the airplane scene. It was fucking frightening. Everyone seemed so advanced, and also so
devoted. My body could, by now, do a lot of things, but this
wasn't going to happen. I simply couldn't see myself tango-
spinning with a partner out of triad.

So I went over and rolled up my mat. The leader looked
at me quizzically. I said, "I'm not comfortable, I'm sorry." He
seemed cool with that. I bowed to him, and left the room.

The teenaged me would have loved those trust-building
exercises. But life and spy novels had taught me, for certain,
that no one could truly be trusted. I felt comfortable in that
knowledge, and in myself, and therefore in my yoga. Then I
realized something. I hadn't *stormed* out or otherwise called
attention to myself; I'd been respectful to the people who
actually *liked* AcroYoga. This, to me, represented promise
for my best self.

Next I went somewhere familiar: the Mysore room.
This was being led by a number of Ashtanga masters, including Nikki Doane and Eddie Modestini, who were out
of rock-star mode and into quiet-yoga-helper mode, where
they seemed very much at ease. I opened the door and saw
that everyone on the floor had a flushed, desperate expression on their face. The air was 50 percent sweat vapor.

I took my blue rectangle, did a few sun salutations, and
then Doane said, "two-minute warning to *savasana!*"

Oh no! I wasn't going to finish my practice! What
would I do? I went over to one of the leaders, who stood
calmly in the back of the room with his arms crossed
behind his back. He had a straight spine and effortlessly
fabulous hair, kind of like the yoga version of late-era
Richard Chamberlain.

"I got here a little late," I said, "and I wasn't able to finish my routine. Any suggestions?"

He tilted his head slightly, like a superior alien life form studying the curiosity that is human behavior. His look said: You can't be serious? But when he saw that I was, in fact, serious, he said to me, kindly:

"Just do *padmasana* and *anjali mudra* and a little *pranayama* and then go into *savasana*."

For the non-Sanskrit speakers, this translates as, "sit in lotus position, hold your hands at your heart, practice breathing, and then rest."

"It's a great opportunity to do nothing," he said.

I had found my teacher.

As fortune would have it, I was actually scheduled to take my next class, Core Mudras and Other Essential Tricks, with the same superior life form, who turned out to be Richard Freeman from Boulder, Colorado. Something about the phrase "essential tricks" grabbed me. Also, a good friend of mine who lives in Boulder swore by the quality of Freeman's yoga, and by the integrity of The Yoga Workshop, the studio he'd founded. In addition to being a physical master of the Ashtanga yoga system, Freeman is also a scholar of Eastern religion, deeply versed in Hindu mythology, Vipassana Buddhism, and Sufi mysticism. His official biography, which is too modest by a degree of at least ten, describes him as "an avid student of Eastern and Western philosophy, as well as Sanskrit." His most prominent work, a multi-CD set called *The Yoga Matrix*, presents a comprehensive view of the Sanskrit chants, breathing techniques, "moral precepts" and "cosmic philosophy" that encompass true, traditional yoga practice. It's not gym yoga. My Boulder friend warned that Freeman could be somewhat of an otherworldly presence at times. She's met Freeman a dozen times, but he never seems to know who she is. "He either doesn't recognize me," she told me, "or he recognizes me on some deeper plane that I can't comprehend."

At 10:30 AM, I spread out my mat next to my car-mate Dhyana. She seemed a little puzzled by the conference, referring to it, with some disdain, as a "smorgasbord." You could either find someone amazing, she said, or get trapped in a room with a total lunatic. That was pretty much the roll of the yoga dice. Meanwhile, she said, I should join her and Denise for lunch. They'd made friends with this cool old San Francisco transpersonal psychologist.

"Oh yeah," I said. "I know that dude."

Meanwhile, I waited for Richard Freeman to appear. I actually wasn't sure, at that point, that he was the same guy who'd told me to do nothing. *Oh, please let it be him*, I thought. I'd been waiting a long time to find a teacher who approved of me doing nothing.

Richard Freeman sat down cross-legged in front of us. Yes, it was he, and he didn't disappoint. He didn't give us much of a workout. In fact, we barely moved. But it was a yoga experience unlike any I'd had before. This guy spoke almost entirely in metaphors and wise aphorisms, which he'd punctuate with weird facial gestures, opening his eyes wide and ripping his mouth into a Joker-like rictus. For instance:

"When you return to your *drishdi*, you have to keep your gaze soft. As we practice *asana* and *pranayama*, we're always returning to the core practice of just gazing."

Wide-eyed clown face.

"You should be looking at reality like a newborn deer."

Even wider clown face.

This went on for an hour and a half. I didn't write down anything he said; I was so consumed watching his gestures that I could barely think. All I know is that he talked, for what seemed like half an hour, about the importance of placing the tip of your tongue on the tip of your palate. There's a reflex in your body between the pelvis and the palate, he said. By placing your tongue there, you loosen up the lower body, and it forces you to smile. This, he said, was all contained in the ancient yogic texts.

There were no casual references to Hindu deities here, or calls for a yoga-fueled social revolution, only the words of ancients and a few sacred physical principles that humans have been practicing since the dawn of time. This was the kind of yoga that inspired, that I wanted to practice. My yoga-sense was tingling. It *blew my mind*.

Oh, no, I realized. I'm a yoga fundamentalist. How the hell did that happen?

After class, Dhyana and I waited for our lunch mates in the hotel lobby. Freeman strolled into view, looking both lost and determined.

"We really wanted to thank you for the class. . . ." I said, but he just walked past us and onto the elevator, muttering something to himself.

After that, we went to the Farmer's Market at the Ferry Building, gathered lots of goodies, and found a swath of bird-shit-covered dockside concrete. Dr. Evil, whose real name was Elliott and who kept getting food stuck in his beard, dominated the conversation. In March 1973, he'd been traveling in India and had found his way to Neem

Karoli Baba, the guru of Ram Dass, who'd taught him that the purpose of life is to explore the reality of our divine nature. While in India, Elliott found himself drawn to the teachings of non-duality, which presents the point of view that no individual can ever have knowledge of God or the Self, since we are that very Self for which we are seeking. All this he explained in a mimeographed flyer, of which he kept many copies in his backpack.

Elliott and Dhyana and I sat there for a while in the radiant sun, talking about non-duality, the suppression of the ego, and *Changeling*, starring Angelina Jolie, which Elliott had recently seen and enjoyed very much. Meanwhile, behind us, Denise practiced the Breath of Joy, gazing at herself in the dirty glass wall of an abandoned municipal building. On a Saturday afternoon in San Francisco, we were pretty much the norm.

Afterward, the three of them were going to see a free lecture by a guy who makes statues of Hindu deities. I went along reluctantly. Hinduism, this guy said, was just a construct of the colonial British, who couldn't understand the variety and mystery of Indian spiritual practice. *File that away for the cocktail parties,* I thought. He went on:

"Shiva is the archetype of anyone who's going through radical change. If you embark on change, you have to destroy . . . Most people live life in a circle. And in a circle, the center never changes. Lord Shiva is saying play the game. Life is a dance."

Well, at this stage of the game, the room was hot and overcrowded. I felt massive dehydration approaching. Besides, I had to dance out of there so I could go do some drugs with a friend.

➡

After an evening that involved two marijuana capsules, a not-fun-enough hotel ballroom "trance dance" led by the famous yoga teacher Shiva Rea, MC Yogi rapping about Hanuman the monkey god, and several beers in a North Beach bar that led to Denise from Canada heading off for an exciting sexual dalliance with the commander of a French battleship, I spent much of Sunday supine in the hotel lobby, watching the NFC Championship game.

I did, however, rouse myself for a final Richard Freeman class before I hit the road for home. He called this one The Root of the Tree, and though it was supposed to be about the *mulabhanda,* or pelvic lock, he more or less covered the same material he had the day before. Conferences, he explained, ask you for your topics months before you teach, so you have to come up with something. But it was all the same teaching, he said, so labels didn't really mean much.

After complaining about the lameness of the previous night's teacher's reception, Freeman apologized in advance. "By the time you get to this point in the conference," he said, "everyone's brain is a muddle and nobody knows what they're doing, Unless you think you know what you're doing, and then you start telling people what to do and then before you know it you're on the cover of *Yoga Journal* and then you're really in trouble."

Richard Freeman, I thought, *you're the man.*

In this final session, Freeman talked about the *sahasra,* the seventh primary chakra, which is located at the top of your head. The *sahasra* is often depicted as a giant lotus with one thousand multi-colored petals, arranged into twenty symmetrical layers of fifty petals each. *Sahasra,*

Freeman said, symbolizes detachment from illusion, the ultimate representation of pure consciousness, the knowledge
that one is all and all is one, and other things written on a
Dr. Bronner's soap bottle. In yoga legend, Freeman said, if
you're aligned just right, you can tip your mouth open just
so—he demonstrated the mouth-tipping—and then you
can taste a few drops of the lotus' nectar, as subtle and sweet
as eternity itself. This went so far beyond "put your knee at
a ninety-degree angle" that my mind could barely contain
it all. Richard Freeman, it seemed, held the key to all yoga
secrets. I needed more time with him.

On that promising note of extreme metaphorical ambi-
guity, my yoga conference ended. I went upstairs and gave
goodbye hugs to my yoga pals. Denise had already hopped a
flight back to Canada. Dhyana was staying behind to attend
meditation retreats and, in the ultimate act of yogic sacrifice, to help Elliott clean his apartment. I had to get home.
My family, not to mention my fantasy-sports teams, needed
tending.

In the car, two twenty-ounce Coke Zeros and an enormous artisanal sausage awaited me. As I drove down I-5
alone, yoga ideas shot through my mind like distant stars
heading toward oblivion. I heard chants and little phrases
of knowledge, and, somewhere behind all that, the distant din of a higher plane. For forty-five minutes, at least, I
floated above mundane reality in my mind, until I realized
that I had to pee.

I stopped at a gas station run by the cast of *The Hills
Have Eyes,* and got the restroom key. The door opened to
reveal a half-inch of turd-water, and a gushing, overflowing
john. It smelled like the end of the world in there.

"Ach!" I said. "Oh, God, no."

But I really needed a piss, and there was no adjacent ditch or tree. It would be the sewer or nothing.

The universe was testing me. Could I detach from my mind and see through to the true nature of reality even as liquid shit brushed my feet? As I emptied the contents of my bladder into the restroom's lone functioning urinal, I thought, in the spirit of the Obama inauguration little more than thirty-six hours away: *Yes I can.* The multi-colored lotus was opening its petals for me, ever so subtly, and dripping a few motes of nectar onto my grateful tongue. I tentatively stood, gagging and sighing, in a fetid puddle of roadside toilet poo, and suddenly, everything tasted so sweet.

A True Quality Journey

My progress through the Ashtanga primary series continued
three times a week in Mara's apartment. This kept my brain
and body sharp and relatively disciplined, the yoga equivalent of going to the gym, but I could have translated Proust
into Farsi faster than I was progressing through the Ashtanga
primary series. I found myself thinking: What next? The conference, though intermittently annoying, had left me itchy for
more.

My first thought, which actually happened months before
I went to the conference, was that I should travel to Mysore,

India, the birthplace of Ashtanga yoga, the seedbed of the practice that had become an unmovable pillar in my life. I'd heard that Patthabi Jois was dying. This would probably be my last chance to study with him.

The Ashtanga Institute's website said that I'd be required to study, at minimum, for a month. That would cost me $500. Additional time would cost additional money. Students had to make their own way to India, of course. While in Mysore, they had to find their own housing and food. That all sounded like big logistical pain in the butt, but I really wanted to practice yoga authentically. So I downloaded an application form and sent it away. That was in June.

Well, now I was going to India. At least I assumed that; they wouldn't turn down my money, right? But as soon as I sent it off, paying, against my will, a certified-mail fee, I began to backslide in my mind. For two months, questions gnawed at me. Did I really want to rent an apartment in Mysore or live by myself in a hotel? Was it truly my destiny to practice yoga in the morning and then spend the rest of my day taking cooking lessons or poking around in ayurvedic-healing shops? Was I that guy? I mean, I wanted to study yoga and all, but an extended pilgrimage to India seemed like something for singles, child-free couples, or people with grown children, an activity for people in transition, not me. I walked around telling people, "I'm going to Mysore," but I did so without enthusiasm in my eyes. The prospect of six weeks in India without my wife and son just didn't appeal to me. The final blow came when I looked at the cost of plane tickets to Bangalore. Five minutes later, I wrote the Ashtanga Institute a letter.

Dear Sirs,

I recently sent an application to study at the Ashtanga Institute in Mysore next January and February. Unfortunately, my financial circumstances don't allow me to travel to India at this time, so I must withdraw my application. I hope to be able to visit next fall instead, and I'll send in a new application at that time. If this has caused you any inconvenience, I sincerely apologize. Thanks for your time.

Namaste,
Neal Pollack
Los Angeles, CA

While it may have been misleading for me to plead "financial circumstances" as a reason for not going, it was probably preferable to expounding upon my *mishegas* about missing my family and my feelings about yoga tourism as a subtle form of colonial exploitation. In any case, I'm sure the Institute was heartbroken. Now they'd have only 399 students instead of 400 in the fall.

My next thought was: *I'll become a licensed yoga teacher.* In the United States, that means going through a Yoga Alliance-approved school. Participating Yoga Alliance studios are called Registered Yoga Schools, or RYS, and people who finish the programs are Registered Yoga Teachers, or RYTs. The standards for RYS are pretty general. The Alliance doesn't care what style of yoga you teach, as long as individual members pay their $55 annual fee. Training requires one hundred hours, minimum, of Techniques

Teaching/Practice, twenty-five of Teaching Methodology, twenty of Anatomy/Phisiology, thirty hours of Yoga Philosophy/Lifestyle and Ethics, ten hours of practice teaching, and fifteen wild-card hours with which the school can fill with whatever crap it wants. Following this, there are another set of requirements if you want to be qualified to teach at the Yoga Alliance five-hundred-hour level. The Alliance also has a somewhat labored and generalized Code of Conduct.

Clearly, though, the Alliance has consumed American yoga, with 964 Registered Yoga Studios from coast to coast. If you want to teach, you'd better join the Yoga Allies. Of course, this begs the question: What are the non-allied teachers? The Yoga Axis? If you don't join the Yoga Alliance, are you Yoga Jong Il?

Los Angeles boasted many Alliance members, including Karuna Yoga, where I'd been attending classes and volunteering for years. If nothing else, Karuna's was one of the most reasonably priced trainings around. I knew several excellent teachers who'd been through that particular mill. But if I was going to spend two hundred hours hanging around a yoga studio, I wanted it to be a different one. Karuna's training was partly *kundalini*-based, and *kundalini* just wasn't for me. Also, I just needed to be in a different room for a while.

Really, if I was going to certify as a yoga teacher in L.A., I would go through Yogaworks. That's where Mara got certified, and Prabhu Prakash, and many other teachers who I liked and respected. Yes, Yogaworks may have been a chain, but at least it was a chain in the Krishnamarcharya lineage. The classes I'd taken there had been too crowded, but there's no denying that the practices had some authenticity and integrity. If I trained at Yogaworks, I'd come out knowing what I was doing.

I made a call, and within two days, had a ten-page multi-colored brochure in my hands for Yogaworks' Yoga Alliance Registered teacher training programs. It had a light-green cover with rows of polka dots. Inside the dots were nature scenes, or shots of people in poses, or portraits of people looking serenely happy, thoughtful, and healthy, a Brave New Yoga World.

This training program, said the brochure, had produced "some of the most celebrated modern-day yogis," and the programs are offered year-round and worldwide, "so you can always find a training to suit your schedule." It was a serious training for serious people, or at the very least, they offered fun Weekend Immersion "retreats-at-home." Along the bottom of the pages ran a Yoga Works timeline, which for the first half was mostly a list of famous graduates, but then it started, around 2004, to chronicle Yogaworks' path toward world domination, ending with 2009: "YWTT in thirty cities, ten countries, and four continents. Soon, no one will be able to stop us, bwah-hah-hah-hah-hah!"

On Page seven, the brochure featured a photograph of an impossibly hot Indonesian-American woman, fully made-up like no one I'd ever seen in a yoga class, bending backwards with Eagle arms. On the top of the page was her testimonial: "On the whole, my spirit was filled with breath, attention, and rejuvenation. It would be very accurate to say yoga—and particularly the teacher training—have made life a true quality journey to walk on and share with." Apparently, the teacher training hadn't covered the dangers of ending sentences with a preposition.

There were also various schedules and teacher-trainer biographies and an application form for me to submit along with a non-refundable $500 deposit. *All right,* I thought. *I will train to become a yoga teacher.* I chose a twelve-weekend intensive at the Center for Yoga on Larchmont, because there was no way in hell I was going to drive all the way out to Pacific Palisades three nights a week. Maybe I'd train in the Palisades when I could actually afford to live in the Palisades, but not a moment before. But then, I didn't send in my application.

A few things were delaying the process for me. The $3,500 fee was in-state college tuition money. They offered a couple of indentured servitude slots, where I'd pay half-price while volunteering many hours at the studio, but that seemed unlikely, given that I had a family and a drug habit to support. In general, the costs didn't compute. Did I really want to pay more than three grand so I could be certified to teach yoga at the YMCA?

Also, I was getting some resistance on the home front.

"You're going to be gone every weekend day for *three months*?" Regina said.

"Only from noon to five," I said. "Plus commute time."

"That's a lot of weekends."

"It's a serious commitment."

"I'm a yoga widow," she said, again.

My wife would survive, but my kid was another story. We were about to sign him up for tee-ball, and this teacher training would take up a season's worth of Saturdays. He didn't seem thrilled at the prospect.

"You're going to be gone *every* weekend?" he said.

"I'll be home for breakfast and dinner," I said.

"What about lunch?"

"Probably not lunch."

"But I *like* eating lunch with you."

Oh, he was laying it on hard.

"We can eat lunch when the training is over."

"What about Father's Day?" he asked.

"Um," I said. "I think that's the last day of training."

"Oh, daddy, no!" Elijah said. "You can't do yoga on Father's Day!"

This kid was making me feel like a neglectful parent for wanting to become a yoga teacher. But he won the day because he was right. I threw the brochure into a drawer with all the other crap I throw into a drawer.

Immediately, I knew I'd chosen well. A Yogaworks teacher-training would have been great for me if I'd been a twenty-five-year-old single woman who possessed both family money and an unquenchable desire to heal the world. But I was pushing forty, married, and financially uncomfortable. Plus, every time I tried to heal anything, someone usually ended up getting hurt.

What I really wanted to do, I realized, was to study more with Richard Freeman. He was, undoubtedly, the smartest and most interesting teacher I'd encountered. For *his* teacher training, I'd walk at least a mile barefoot, assuming it wasn't too hot outside. So I went to his website. His training, while not exactly dime-store priced, cost about two-thirds of YogaWorks. The only drawbacks: He only gave one a year, they lasted a full month, and they took place in Boulder.

"So," I said to Regina, "What would you think about me studying in Boulder for a month?"

"Would you have to move there?"

"Probably."

"Would that month be July or August?"

"November."

"Then the answer is no."

Again, practical concerns—like the fact that I'd be leaving for my family for a month to sublet a room in Boulder—trumped yoga desires. I started looking for a more short-term fix. Like all high-end yoga teachers, Richard Freeman had a pretty cool traveling schedule. The website said that, in 2009, he'd be teaching for a week in London and a week in Greece, both appealing destinations for sure, but a week seemed awfully short. The same went for a week in Taiwan. There was a four-day thing in Istanbul around the same time as the Greece workshop, and I really wanted to go to Istanbul, but if I wouldn't do a week, then why do four days?

The best choice seemed to be a two-week Richard Freeman retreat at a yoga center in Thailand. As soon as I saw that listed, I knew that was where my destiny lay. I hadn't pushed anything else very hard with Regina, probably because I really hadn't wanted to do anything else very much. But this one smelled like a winner to me.

I went downstairs, where my wife was making jewelry at her desk.

"Hey, guess where I'm gonna go?" I said.

"Where?"

"Thailand."

"Can I come?"

"Only if you want to do hard-core Ashtanga yoga for two weeks in a tropical climate."

"You bastard," she said.

No contemporary yoga experience can be considered complete without a retreat. Every teacher worth his or her incense burner has one, and they don't just take place in India or Bali. Thousands of centers, either full- or part-time, have appeared all over the world, in such traditional yogic locales as Playa del Carmen, Peru, Maui, and Maine. Take some pounding surf adjacent to a quiet, contemplative forest or jungle, add a breakfast buffet, and yoga people are sure to follow with their mats and checkbooks.

Nothing can really justify my descent into yoga tourism. I had a teacher, and I wanted to follow him. He happened to be offering a course at a retreat center in Thailand. As prices for such things went, this one was pretty good. I'd done a little comparative shopping. A week in Mexico with a run-of-the-mill *anusara* teacher cost about the same as two weeks in Asia with the smartest, humblest, coolest yoga teacher I'd ever encountered.

But I wouldn't exactly call the retreat a *bargain*. Paying for it required . . . you know what? Fuck it. Here's how I managed: I had a portion of my advance yet to be paid for this book. It wasn't an enormous amount of money, but it was enough. My publisher forwarded me a fraction of that amount, and I wired that money to Thailand. Plus, my father had a lot of frequent-flier miles on British Airways. He'd recently gotten soaked in the economic downturn. As he put it, "I'm not going to be using those miles any time soon." So he scored me an economy ticket to Bangkok, by way of Hong Kong. From there, I had to make my way, on a puddle-jumper, to Koh Samui, the island where the retreat would be going down.

Yes, I was a thirty-nine-year-old American man flying to a yoga retreat in Asia, without my family, on daddy's frequent-flier miles. This made me one of the most loathsome creatures in the world. I understood this. But I'd wired the money, and secured the travel documents. Nothing could stop me from going now.

Except, possibly, political unrest. You may remember, or not, that Thailand has had some problems in recent years. The Thai military seized control of the country in 2006, booting out the leader, Thaksin Shinawatra, who they accused of running Thailand as a criminal front for his telecom empire. Then Thaksin came back in 2008 to try to rescue some of his frozen assets. That lasted a few months, until he returned, because of "security threats," to exile in England, where he owned the Manchester City football club. Perhaps from his owner's box, he began issuing calls for a people's revolution, and the battles began. The military had their supporters, who wore a certain color shirt. Thaksin had his supporters, who wore different-colored shirts. The military people seized the airport. Thaksin's supporters started throwing bombs during an economic summit. The rural poor continued, as always, to live in wretchedness. Travelers from more stable countries, myself included, began thinking that maybe they should stay away from this god-awful mess.

I sent an email to the retreat center:

"Hi there," I wrote. "I'm scheduled to visit Richard Freeman's workshop in June. Naturally, I'm concerned about the political violence in Thailand right now. I realize that it doesn't affect your part of the country directly at the moment, and may never, but there are rumors of the situation spreading. Will you all be keeping us posted? If I decide that I don't feel comfortable visiting Thailand during the political strife, can I get a full or partial refund? Sorry to bother you with this, but I'm sure you understand. Thanks so much."

They got back to me the same day:

"Thank you for your email. We can understand your concern about Thailand's political situation. The situation seems to be under control now and we hope it will be better this week. The protests do not affect us in Koh Samui and will not spread here based on past experiences in dealing with this. We are an hour flight from Bangkok and everything is normal here. Koh Samui is a tourist travel destination without any national government bodies represented. The protestors are mainly at the Bangkok national government sites.

As we did last December 2008 with the protest situation, we will be happy to keep your full payment as credit to be used at Yoga Thailand without an expiration time if you choose to postpone your trip."

In other words: You're coming, sucker.

As I moved through May, preparations for my big trip began to accelerate. I secured vital supplies of mosquito repellent, Immodium, and, most important, Xanax. I wasn't about to fly for thirteen hours without soporific aid. Regina, with the realization setting in that she'd be taking care of a six-year-old for two weeks without any help, kept me fully apprised of the rocky Thai political situation, hoping that I'd change my mind. In early May, a couple of young female tourists, one American, one Norwegian, died horribly of a mysterious ailment at resorts in the same archipelago where I'd be staying. Regina made sure to send me news accounts of their autopsy reports.

Then, on May 18, ten days before I was due to leave for Thailand, a friend sent me this email, a forward of a forward:

"Dear Students of Ashtanga Yoga," it read, "Our Beloved Guru Ji, Sri Krishna Patthabi Jois, has passed this morning. Blessings to a great man who has given our planet much greatness in his time. It is amazing the wealth that he has contributed in his lifetime. I am extremely grateful for his hard work and devotion to all of us, Ashtanga Yoga, and to God. We are so fortunate to have had a great Guru bless us and give us strength and truth."

Oh, how very sad. The world had lost one of its most influential yoga teachers. One could very easily argue that yoga as we know it today wouldn't exist without Patthabi Jois. The annoying things about yoga culture definitely aren't his fault. He gave us yoga's best face: discipline, strength, intelligence, and, best of all, a sense of humor. I'm writing as though I knew him, which, of course, I didn't. But when I heard about his death, I felt incredibly grateful to him for his yoga, which had made my life better in profound ways.

So when I received an email the next day informing me that there would be a memorial service for Guru Ji at the Ashtanga Shala in Silverlake, I knew that I should attend. There was one problem, though: I had Dodger tickets for that night, and they were playing the Mets, which doesn't happen that often. I called the friend who'd forwarded me the email, and related my dilemma. She wasn't sympathetic.

"Don't you think there will be plenty of mourning in Thailand?" I said.

"Justify it however you want," she said. "But you know you should go."

She was right, of course, and the shala *was* right down the street from Dodger Stadium. Still, with a 6 PM service and a 7:10 first pitch, I'd be shaving it awfully close. I called my friend Jerod, who'd be going with me to the game. Jerod had done yoga, but only Iyengar, and not for a while.

"So before the game I need to go to a memorial service for the founder of Ashtanga yoga," I said.

"Oooo-kaaaaaay," he said.

"So I kind of feel like I have to go. You can stay in the car if you want."

"No way, dude," he said. "I'm going. *And I'm gonna wear my Dodgers jersey.*"

"Just don't be disrespectful," I said.

When we got there, Jerod's Dodgers' jersey made me nervous.

"I'd prefer if you took that off," I said.

"Why?"

"It's just too flashy."

"And my T-shirt isn't?" he said.

His T-shirt featured a black-and-white image of pre-suspension Manny Ramirez, in street clothes, and the word "Legend" written underneath. I had one, too. We'd bought them for ten bucks off a vendor right after Manny got traded to the Dodgers.

"Nah," I said. "They'll just think it's Bob Marley."

We went upstairs. A man and a woman, each bearing a gaze of sweet sympathetic sadness, were holding copper pots.

They dipped their hands in and daubed our foreheads. We got a yellow schmear, followed by a smaller red schmear. As we sat down, Jerod whispered, "we've got to wipe these off before the game, or we're going to get our asses kicked."

About thirty people were sitting cross-legged on the floor. On the wall were a series of lovely photos of Guru Ji himself, as a younger man, demonstrating his Ashtanga poses to their full expression. The woman who'd sent me the email sat down next to us.

"So what's with the schmears?" I asked.

"I don't know. You get them anywhere you go in India. Something to do with mourning," she said.

"That much, I'd figured out," I said.

She practiced here regularly.

"It's a nice room," Jerod said.

"Yeah, well, you're not here at nine in the morning when it's full of a thousand sweaty, disgusting people," she said.

"True enough," he said.

Then they talked about *American Idol* for a while until the priest showed up. He mumbled something incomprehensible in English, and then began somber devotional chanting in Sanskrit. The room followed along. I just observed. After about five minutes, Jerod and I looked at each other, and the clock. We bolted the room, each grabbing a tissue to wipe off our schmear. Outside, he said to me,

"You got red stuff on your nose. How do I look?"

"Like you dipped your forehead in mustard," I said. "Perfect for the ballgame."

"Dude," he said. "That wasn't yoga. That was *religion*."

"Duh," I said. "Though I would term it more spirituality than religion. Yoga and Hinduism share a lot of philosophy and texts, and there's also a huge intersection with Buddhism, but yoga is, technically, not tied to any one religion."

"Still," he said.

"I know," I said.

"I just like doing the poses."

"That's what I used to say."

The next day, I got an email from my friend: "You didn't miss much yesterday. About a half hour of chanting and then people started telling these long-winded tales of their time with guru ji . . . at which point I bailed."

Meanwhile, the Dodgers had won, 5–3, on a three-run shot by Casey Blake late in the game. The next morning, like thousands of other members of the cult of Ashtanga, I went to practice. Guru Ji may have been gone, but he'd left us with six series of near-impossible yoga poses that were going to torment us for the rest of our lives. Sometimes, we were even grateful for them.

15

At the Feet of the Dude-Ji

The moon shone over placid high-tide waters. Gentle breezes whispered through the coconut palms. The night murmured with the faint sounds of recorded *kirtan*. It was Saturday, nearly twenty-four hours before the program would begin. I sat at a table in the *sattva,* or dining area, of Yoga Thailand, with a half-dozen Austrians, trying to keep them amused.

The two Xanax I'd taken the previous night (or morning, or maybe two nights previous), still buzzed through my brain in trace amounts. I'd given myself a day on the front end so I could adjust to the jet lag, but that obviously wasn't going to be enough. The Austrians spoke perfect English, but when they opened their mouths I barely understood what they were saying. It took all my mental strength not to do a face-plant into my supper.

"You're not doing yourself justice unless you leave here with a Yoga Thailand cookbook," one of them said.

They couldn't get enough of the buffet, included in the cost of the program: black bean soup, "Spanish" corn, zucchini grilled with peppers, all of it blander than anything I'd find on my local mid-range grocery store steam table. The only thing Thai about the meal, as far as I could discern, was the lemongrass they gave you to soak in your hot water.

I said something to this effect.

"You don't like the food?" someone responded.

I decided to keep quiet for the moment. It was too early in the experience to make enemies; that could wait for the second week. Instead, yoga experiences were shared, and the beauty of the place remarked upon. One of the Austrians was celebrating a birthday, and they'd ordered a cake. The staff brought out a flourless, desiccated brown disc, with some fruit. That wouldn't do, said the Austrians. Where was the *schlag*? You can't have cake without *schlag*. One of them went back into the kitchen, to demand some.

"I had to *schlag* through three airports just to get here," I said.

No one laughed.

I fell asleep long before 9 PM, my head throbbing with weird, low echoes. Around 4:30 AM, I woke. My back hurt and my bones felt cold. Had I turned the air conditioner down too low? Had I remembered to hydrate? Was that really a neon portrait of Bob Marley's face hanging over my bed? I couldn't answer those questions when I'd gone to bed, and I still couldn't.

Totally naked and not very clean, I wrenched myself out of bed and walked onto my enclosed porch. I beheld wondrous jungle verdure and a glistening pool, subtly lit, encircled by beach chairs and umbrellas. Beyond that, I could see a restaurant, and a pavilion offering free twenty-four-hour Internet. I heard roosters and the occasional moped.

Wait, this wasn't Yoga Thailand. Where the hell was I?

Oh, yes, I sort of remembered. I'd signed up for the Richard Freeman program late. They didn't have room at the yoga center. Instead, I was being housed at the auxiliary hotel, three minutes up the road. For the next two weeks, I would be living at the evocatively named Easy Time Resort.

Holy shit, I realized.

I'm on vacation.

For some reason, that hadn't occurred to me before.

In Alex Garland's novel *The Beach*, Koh Samui is where the backpackers travel on their way to an untouched island paradise. In other words, Samui was already over when he published that book, more than a decade ago. By the time I got to there, it had become South Padre Island with a Muay Thai stadium and live elephant shows.

The founders of Yoga Thailand, strong devotees of Patthabi Jois, opened their Ashtanga-inspired shala in the early aughts, on the northern side of the island, a short *tuk-tuk* ride from the disco beer-bar nightmare that is Chaweng Beach. As the years passed, the area got even less yoga-friendly. But apparently, the center did pretty well, because a few years later, the owners built *another* center, on the less-populated southern shore, in an area dominated by homes for the wealthy. Let me now quote from the promotional materials:

"Situated on Laem Sor beach, Yoga Thailand is surrounded by towering coconut trees in a quiet, spacious area, with incredible sunrises and sets that play with the colors of the water, sand and greenery. Only a few hundred meters away is the well-known Laem Sor Pagoda, which houses the remains of Leung Poo Daeng, a realized monk. The only other structures in the area are villas privately owned. As such, our beach is private and virtually undisturbed. With the main shopping areas still within easy reach, about fifteen to thirty minutes away by car or motorbike, Yoga Thailand has a peaceful setting that inspires long, refreshing walks either on the beach or the meandering back roads."

Those are all pluses. On the negative side, a sign at the entrance of Yoga Thailand indicates that alcohol and drugs are strictly prohibited. They allow caffeinated drinks, but they're not included with meals and must be ordered a la carte.

Perhaps on the strength of such financial calculations, Yoga Thailand has constructed a yoga temple in the jungle, with stark white walls, slate walkways, and dark wood everywhere. Behind the open-air reception desk, a stunning, bright red wall features the Ashtanga practice's closing chant, written in bright yellow letters in all four corners, one in Sanskrit, one Thai, one transliteration, and one in plain English. Next to the reception desk is a gift shop and boutique, selling plastic water bottles for 710 *baht* (more than twenty bucks), as well as lots of pink clothing bearing the Yoga Thailand logo, and, for a few bucks, a laminated brochure depicting the studio owner doing Ashtanga poses.

Heading toward the water, you pass the "wellness center" and its various massage rooms, a smoothie-and-coffee bar, and the aforementioned *sattva,* which has two levels, one with conventional tables and wicker chairs and an upper area of cushions and row tables for dining Thai-style.

Then there's the shala itself, three rooms of wood-floored yoga heaven, sweetly decorated with photos of revered teachers, art depicting scenes from Indian mythology, and little shrines to deities whose lineages go over the heads of most of the patrons, including me. The shala has no air-conditioning, but does contain powerful fans, as well as floor-to-ceiling glass windows on three walls. These open with a simple crank. Behind where the teacher sits, at the front of the room, are various closets full of props, cushions, and, in a sure sign that this is a serious house of yogic instruction, anatomical skeletons.

The studio overlooks a calm inlet where longboats bob, just offshore, waiting for an errand or a commission. Behind them, in the not-too-far distance, are several islands, apparently unpopulated, except, perhaps, by Leonardo DiCaprio and his secret group of friends. Also in view: a small but pleasant pool, and an herbal steam room, free in the evenings, with portholes designed to overlook the sea.

In all, Yoga Thailand makes a lovely spot for a man to stagger into at five in the morning.

No one else was around except a security guard, who was watching a portable TV, and his dog. They both ignored me, obviously used to the sight of dazed, recently arrived

Westerners bumping into walls at dawn like a yoga version of Edmund O'Brien at the end of *D.O.A.* My head felt
wicked and weird, my chest and nose gummy. The earth
undulated beneath me, as though I didn't belong on its surface. Not only had I never been to Thailand before, I'd never
been to *Asia* before. My body obviously didn't appreciate
this massive shift in time and space.

A hammock hung between two coconut trees. There
I lay for forty-five minutes, waiting for the sun, trying to
breathe away the bad feelings gathering around my gills. At
some point, apparently, I got up, because the next thing I
could remember, I was reclining on some cushions, having
a friendly conversation with a yoga-studio owner from
Portland whose husband plays in the Dandy Warhols. Well,
we had a lot in common then, I said. I was in a band too,
once. We put out one album and toured for nearly three
weeks. She seemed vaguely interested.

At some point, as she talked, I grabbed my temples and
said,

"Ohhhhhhhh."

"Are you all right?" she said.

"I think I have allergies."

"You could be dehydrated."

"What did you just say?"

My ears had begun to hum. There was movement in the
shala. The Richard Freeman workshop hadn't begun yet,
but Yoga Thailand offered a regular Mysore-style practice,
guided by staff members.

"I think I'm going to start practicing," she said.

I nodded as I blew my nose, hard, into a napkin.

For a little while, I lay there, murmuring to myself. Suddenly, my headache grew unbearable. My eyes began to roll around. The avalanche approached. I tore off my sleeveless shirt, ran for the bathroom, and reached the toilet just in time to yarf up my guts. Three massive heaves later, I didn't feel any better. Usually, that does the job. Man, Asia gave me some *nasty* allergies.

Despite the fact that I'd just massively upchucked the two bananas that I'd eaten before I left my hotel, I decided that now would be a good time for me to practice. So I went into the shala, making sure to daub the vomity bits off my chest, and unrolled my mat. Outside, the air already felt milky-thick and breezeless. Inside, it was desperately, unbearably, ass-scorching hot. The moisture poured off me as though my skin were the staging area for a monsoon. I needed windshield wipers for my eyes. Sweat pooled in my nostrils, ears, and belly button. My head felt strange and light. At one point, I forgot how to do a pose that I'd figured out years before. I called the instructor over.

"Yeah, um," I said, "you know the one after the forward fold where you're supposed to thrust your hips upward?"

"*Purvattasana*," she said.

"Yeah, that one," I said. "How do you do that again?"

"So much to remember," she said.

Just show me the pose, lady, I thought.

At last, my practice finished. I'd done pretty much the whole thing, as far as I was able. During *savasana*, bugs danced inside my brain. It was the least-relaxing corpse pose ever. I walked outside. The air smelled like nasty steamed vegetables. Brunch was nearly upon us.

I went up the stairs and lay on a cushion, moaning. At some point, I must have fallen asleep, and then again, because twice I woke myself up with the sound of my own snoring. Then I sat up. People were starting to drift out of practice toward the steam tables. A woman sat down across from me. I got a whiff of the food. To me, it *reeked*.

"Ohhhhh," I moaned.

"What's the matter?" she said.

"Don't feel so good," I said.

"You should have a coconut," she said.

That was a good idea, but coconuts weren't on the all-inclusive menu.

I felt incontrovertibly, violently nauseated. This time, I couldn't get my shirt off, and though I somehow reached the bathroom, I didn't make it to the toilet. Instead, I leaned over the sink, and I was loud.

"BLEARGH!" I said.

From the ladies' room, across the way, I heard someone say, "Oh my!"

One of that morning's practice leaders walked into the bathroom.

"Are you OK?" she asked.

"BLEARGH!" I said.

A shower of clear liquid erupted from my mouth and spattered the counter.

"Oh my!" she said again.

Had I unwittingly undergone a yoga exorcism?

At some point, my insides had nothing left to give. She patted my mouth with a wet wipe, took me outside, and sat me at a table. Understandably, she looked concerned. I wanted to explain to her that I wasn't actually sick, just prone to melodramatic vomiting, but I couldn't form the words just then.

"Do you need to go to hospital?" she asked, in a kind Liverpool accent.

"No," I said. "It's not viral."

She summoned the staff nurse, who quickly appeared bearing some sort of orangey electrolyte solution. I gulped it down very quickly. The nurse brought me another, which I also gulped. Along came two of my fellow workshop attendants, an Irish doctor and a Colombian doctor who were currently dating and practicing in Darwin, Australia. They determined that I was just jet-lagged and dehydrated. I needed to eat just a little food. A piece of dry toast arrived. This I devoured like a coyote eating a jackrabbit. Suddenly, I was starving. I approached the buffet omnivorously, ravenously, and heaped my plate high with brown rice, and toast, and eggs, and made myself the biggest bowl of granola with soy milk possible. This surprised everyone who'd been attending to me. Five minutes previous, I'd been showing all the symptoms of a mid-stage malaria patient.

"Are you sure you should be eating that much?" said my new Irish doctor friend.

"Oh yeah," I said, my mouth full of eggs. "I'll be fine."

As I walked back very slowly toward the Easy Time Resort, I felt surprisingly good. My body had purged itself, and now my mind felt fresh and pure as well. For the next two weeks, I had nothing in front of me but fresh experience. Even my miseries, and they were numerous indeed, would be enjoyable. No amount of puke, or heat, or annoyingly bland vegetarian food could keep me from my appointed rounds. All felt new, and bright, and alive. Before I'd even seen the teacher, my yoga transformation was underway.

➡

Finally, more than twenty-four hours after I'd arrived, and nearly twelve after I'd vomited for the first time, the teacher held a session. Richard had been hovering around the edges since I'd gotten there, swooping in for a quick, near-silent dinner, and an even stealthier breakfast. I understood why he'd want to make those visits short. It was possible that he didn't want to sit with a bunch of strangers who were sitting around talking about the quality of their breath, or maybe he just felt shy. Regardless, at 5:30 PM on Sunday, he said hello.

He'd just come from Mysore, and it had been strange and sad, but he was glad he'd paid homage to his *guruji*. Today, he told us, marked the fourteenth day since the death of Patthabi Jois. At this very moment, he said, the city of Mysore was holding a great banquet for many thousands of people. "They can finally let him go," he said. As I watched the Yoga Thailand staff set up the steam tables for that night's vegetarian buffet, I found myself thinking longingly about the Mysore festival food.

Now, Richard said, we should introduce ourselves. So we went around the shala. Eight or nine people came from Vienna. Taiwan also had a large contingent. The third most-represented country was the United States, but there were also delegates from Denmark, Holland, Finland, Argentina, Costa Rica, Canada, Singapore, Japan, and many other fine nations. In all, twenty countries could boast representatives. We were a truly international coalition of yoga nerds.

Everyone gave a little sentence on the subject of "why are you here?" That seemed like a logical question. Mostly, they answered, "because I want to study with Richard."

One of the Austrian dudes said that he'd illegally down-loaded Richard's audiobook, *The Yoga Matrix*, and that this was his way of paying Richard back.

I stood up and said, "Hi, my name's Neal, and I'm from Vienna, Austria." A few confused chuckles came from the group. "No, no," I said. "Actually, I'm from L.A. I took a couple of classes from Richard at a conference, and his were the only ones I really liked, so I decided to travel seven thousand miles to study with him."

From there, Richard outlined the two-week program. Every day from 7 to 10 AM, or maybe until 10:30, we'd have *asana* class, or physical yoga. Then, there'd be a long break. At 3:30, we'd reconvene to study the *Yoga Sutras*, do some breathing exercises, learn some chanting, and prac-tice meditation. This would run until 6 PM, and then the evenings were our own to stare at the ocean while gently wiping the drool from our mouths, the only action we'd be able to execute after six hours of practicing yoga in a brutal, steamy tropical climate.

And so, the next morning, it began. We lined up our mats, wall to wall, front to back, sixty of us in total, leav-ing not a single space unoccupied. The staff, also eager to practice with the master, overflowed onto the walkway. All non-kitchen activity at the resort stopped, except for the yoga practice. The air felt still, sometimes too still, the only noises coming from barking dogs, the occasional truck driving down a dirt road, or the ominous clanging of dishes announcing another under-seasoned buffet.

Yoga was about to happen.

Richard began leading us through simple poses, all while talking more than I'd ever heard a yoga teacher talk.

That first day, the subject was *prana*, the energy force that activates yoga poses during the inhalation of breath, and *apana,* the exhalation, the relaxing breath, the cooling of the life force. In one of his favorite metaphors, used over and over again during the course of the two weeks, Richard likened the *prana* and *apana* to lovers separated for all eternity but forever seeking each other. One leaves just as the other arrives, leading to great disappointment but followed by the great hope, carried by both lovers, that they'll eventually meet. Their tragic desire, somewhat movingly brought to life in the 1980s fantasy movie *Ladyhawke,* equals our breath.

Speaking of breath, Richard said, as we raised our arms above our heads with dignity, we needed to relax our soft palate to help along the sacred sound of the *ujaii.* If done properly, this should have the effect of releasing you from your brain's control, making you, in effect, an idiot.

He did one of his wacky facial contortions, complete with eye roll.

"That's all the breath is," he said. "The wind blowing around inside of an idiot."

Thus began a streak of Richard uttering the greatest things I'd ever heard in yoga class. At one point, he referred to the *mulabahnda,* the space between the pubic bone and the coccyx that serves as the root of all yoga poses, as the "golden poo." He continually talked about how energy moves through the body during practice, and that it should exit the head sharply, a move he called "vomiting out of the head." This was yoga done right.

Often, he'd go off on wondrous philosophical tangents. He talked about how obsessed some people are with perfecting the postures, "to the point where they'd sell their soul to Satan to perfect them. In return, all Satan would want is the center of their heart, and also for them to burn in hell for eternity."

"Here, Satan," he said, extending his hand. "Take it. There's nothing there anyway."

Then he did a perfect seated bound half-lotus pose, or, more accurately, he parodied a person getting into one. When he got there, he said, with a bit of a hiss,

"And now you're certified."

We loved that so much, we applauded.

That class laid me flat on my ass, my jet-lagged brain bouncing with all of his bizarre turns of phrase. Then, after a busy break of brunching and bobbing around in the pool and drinking coconut milk, I made the steamy walk from Easy Time to the yoga place, for the *sutras* portion of the day. This was the part that I'd been anticipating. I was finally about to dive into the roots of yoga philosophy. My brain would fill with wisdom. At last, I'd *understand*.

We began, somewhat disappointingly, by chanting the vowels of the Sanskrit alphabet. If you're going to chant, Richard told us, you've got to pronounce the words properly. You need to know accent marks and syllable breaks. "If you're in India and chanting," he said, "and you put the accent on the wrong syllable, Sanskrit people look at you funny."

Simple chanting, he explained, was how they taught Sanskrit to kindergarteners in India. Given our level of Sanskrit knowledge, that seemed appropriate. We gazed up at Richard in wonder, like the Muppets dreamily gathering around John Denver during his Christmas special.

He chanted:

"*a aa, e ee, oo oooo,*"

"*a aa, e ee, oo oooo,*" we Sanskrit kindergarteners chanted back.

"*ai I o au um . . . a-ha.*"

"*ai I o au um . . . a-ha.*"

A couple of repetitions of that, and he seemed vaguely satisfied.

Now, at last, we could dig into the *Yoga Sutras*. No one knows exactly when the *sutras* were written, but we do know that they post-date the Buddha, who himself post-dates the ancient Vedic chants that form the soul-core of most yoga philosophy. So yoga and Buddhism, Richard said, were totally intertwined, and had used each other for good and evil, but mostly good, throughout the last two millennia of human existence.

The great sage Patanjali wrote the *Sutras*. In mythology, Richard said, Pantajali was a giant serpent with an infinite number of heads. He would occasionally grow a human torso in order to make himself more accessible to those who wished to study his teachings. This may sound farfetched, but literary history boasts a long tradition of snake-man authors. Norman Mailer would often do the same thing before his readings, and he had a long and prosperous career.

Sutras, in the lovely words of a Swami Sivananda commentary that I found on the Internet, are terse, aphoristic sayings, "pregnant with deep, hidden significance." "A Yogi with full realization can explain the Sutras beautifully," Sivananda writes. "Literally, *sutra* means a thread. Just as various kinds of flowers with different colors are nicely arranged in a string, to make a garland, just as rows of pearls are beautifully arranged in a string to form a necklace, so also Yogic ideas are well arranged in *sutras*."

In all, there are 186 *sutras*, divided into four chapters. Strung together, they outline a complex path, Sivananda says, at the end of which the "Yogi sits at ease, watches his mind and silences the bubbling thoughts. He stills the mind, restrains the thought-waves and enters into the thoughtless state."

As we sat there on a Thai island, Richard Freeman, a fully realized yogi if I'd ever met one, started with the first *sutra*, a very good place to start. He chanted it in Sanskrit, and we chanted back. Then he read it, in English, from the translation we were using:

"Now, the teachings of yoga."

What the hell did that mean?

Richard was kind enough to tell us.

"Finally," he said, "you're coming to the point where you crave liberation, having seen that the other schemes of the mind do not work to relieve suffering."

Yes, I thought.

"For most of us who've been practicing yoga for years, we're actually practicing for the day that we might *start* yoga," he said. All matter, experience, and thoughts are impermanent, and when you grasp the truth of that impermanence in your heart, that's when you truly begin. "You're practicing to start practicing," he said. "It's like renting with an option to buy."

We went on to the second *sutra*, perhaps the most important sentence in all the billions of words that have been written about yoga throughout the eons. It goes, in Sanskrit transliteration:

Yogas citta-vrtti nirodhah

The English translation says "yoga is to still the pattern-ing of consciousness," but Richard was able to explain this vague saying quite clearly. Understanding the word *vritti*, he said, was the key to unlocking this particular mental puzzle. Though *vrtti* technically translated to mean "pat-terning, turning, movements," it could really be applied to anything in our lives. Imagine a *vrtti* as a mosquito buzzing around your head, distracting you from your yoga practice. Mosquitoes were actual *vrttis*, as were thoughts of mosqui-toes. In fact, all thoughts were *vrtti*, both ideas and memo-ries. Anything in the physical world could serve as *vrtti*, as could anything in your head. The world, according to the ancient texts, is a cruel trick played on us by the gods, seek-ing to distract us from the true nature of reality, otherwise known as *isvara*, or pure awareness. Thus we practice yoga to calm the mind and reach the state of *nirodhah*, a stilling of your *citta*, or consciousness, which gets distracted by all these *vrtti*.

The collected *vrtti*, Richard said, create something called *samskara*, an overlaying of negative impressions that only serve to advance suffering. Even happiness is suffering, he said, because it's going to end. If you become too attached to the idea of being happy, then suffering will eventually find you. Yoga is about getting rid of these "negative loops," he said. When that happens, yoga's famous dualism kicks in, and the "seer stands in pure consciousness. The seen is anything that's experienced."

"The thinking process has to stop," he said. "If you're not in the enlightened state, then the seer is in the form of the seen. Everything is in temporary composition. When you look closely, you'll see that whatever you're looking at is purely transformation."

Therefore, he said, you have to be mindful of thoughts, sensations, and identifications. You get rid of the concept of "I" and obliterate the observing intelligence. He used, as an example, a delicious mango *lassi*, which sat by his side every day as he taught us the *sutras*. The *lassi* was so much better, he said, if you enjoyed its unnamable properties, rather than trying to define anything about it. "It's so much more delicious and effervescent," he said. In other words, don't become attached to anything, and you'll be much more content.

This all sounded very interesting to me. But I had some questions. I raised my hand, and he called on me.

"All right," I said. "I understand not wanting to name something good. And I understand using non-attachment to get over grief or a bad relationship. But what if you stub your toe or step in dog poo. How do you get over that?"

"Dog poo?" Richard said.

"Well, discomfort or pain."

He nodded. Basically, he said, you step in the poo. You notice it squish between your toes, acknowledge the feeling, and then you acknowledge the smell, realizing that it's poop instead of just garden-variety mud, and then you deal with the situation. But the important part, he said, is to realize that it has *nothing to do with you,* the perceived self. You shouldn't despair because you stepped in dog poo. The universe has not singled you out for misery. It's just life, in a constant state of transformation.

"Oh, I have been despoiled," he said, sweetly but also sarcastically.

And that's what the *Yoga sutras* teach us about stepping in dog poo.

Not staying at the yoga center itself improved my time enormously. The rooms there had been recently built, and had all the amenities of a modern boutique hotel, minus television, of course. But they also felt a little cold, impersonal, and austere. I guess if you're looking for a wild party atmosphere, don't go to an Ashtanga-themed resort.

The scene at the Easy Time, on the other hand, resembled something out of *La Dolce Vita*. It had a clean, light, relaxing, and fun atmosphere with no secrets and no pretensions. Two half-Italian, half-Algerian brothers ran the hotel and were omnipresent in its operations. One of them, who'd trained at a culinary academy in Italy, guarded the kitchen area, and particularly his pizza oven, like a nervous ocelot wearing a chef's shirt. He was small and clean cut, and could often be found smoking a cigarette and drinking late-night shots by the cash register with various local figures of interest, of both the Thai and expat variety. The other brother was a hulking, tan, tattooed Rastafari who stalked the grounds of the Easy Time, glowering ominously until he saw you, and then he threw off a big, laid-back smile. He often could be seen alongside his wife, a cute Russian blond who couldn't have been older than twenty-five. In the afternoon, he'd take their little blond toddler for a ride on his moped, and the child would scream merrily into the hot wind.

Unsurprisingly, the brothers had different philosophies about how to run the Easy Time day-to-day. Those exact differences remained obscure to their guests, but we could tell they existed, because almost every day, they'd go into a storeroom and scream profanities in Italian for about thirty minutes. Then, it would be quiet for a little while, and they'd come out, literally brothers in arms, and go to the kitchen for a glass of Prosecco. They really knew how to live, these two.

On my second day there, in between Richard's classes, I bobbed around in the pool, occasionally emerging to make half-assed stabs at reading the Paul Bowles novel I'd brought along. At some point, this being vacation and all, I began to think a snack might be nice. I walked into the kitchen area, dripping water. The chef regarded me as though I'd just emerged from the Black Lagoon.

"How're you?" he said.

"I'm fine," I said. "How are you?"

"Eh," he said, waving his hand around in the air. "The so-so."

"Well, anyway, I was wondering if you had *proscuitto y melone*?"

This was, I realized, an atypical request for Thailand, but when in Rome, so to speak, you ask for Roman food.

"Not possible today," he said.

"Oh, no prosciutto available here?"

"No no. Prosciutto no problem. It's the melon. Hard to find melon that's sweet enough."

Totally by accident, I'd walked into my dream hotel. That afternoon, I was strolling back to my room. The Rasta stopped me and shook my hand.

"Hey, Mr. Neal, I like your shirt," he said.

"Oh, thanks."

"Bob Marley is my Jesus," he said.

"OK," I said, and then I realized that he, like so many other people, had mistaken the image of Manny Ramirez on my shirt for that of the great Lion of Zion.

"No, no," I said. "This isn't Bob Marley. He's Manny Ramirez, a cool baseball player who takes steroids."

"Hang on a second," he said. "I get something for you."

So I sat at the reception desk, carefully observing the sweat droplets emanating from my every pore. He returned five minutes later, pressing something into my hand, while murmuring something about the majesty of Emperor Haile Selassie.

"Wow," I said.

"It is a gift from me to you," he said.

"What am I supposed to do with this?" I asked.

"You don't know what to do?" he asked. He looked surprised.

"No, no, I do. Thank you."

"We must perpetuate," he said, and he hulked away.

That night, after a desperate-tasting yoga buffet of sautéed kale, zucchini and peppers, rice pilaf, and vegetarian chili, I got some people to come back to Easy Time with me by uttering the phrase, "Fuck this. Let's go get some wine." Anyone who responded positively to that message, I decided, would be my special yoga friend. One of the people who went back with me ordered a *pizza margherita*, and passed out slices. The sauce tasted perfect and the cheese melted to just the right consistency. The basil was, of course, fresh, and the crust was light, almost cracker-like. My jaw collapsed like a cartoon wolf's. This pizza tasted spectacular. It really did rival the best pizza I'd had in Italy. I went up to the chef, who was smoking by himself next to the cash register.

"Yes?" he said. "How may I help?"

"That pizza was fantastic," I said.

"No good?" he said.

"No, FANTASTIC!" I said. "The best. The best."

"Ah," he said, pointing at his chest, proudly. "Napoli."

"Napoli!" I said. "The birthplace of pizza! Oh, Napoli!"

"Napoli!" he exclaimed, and we embraced like brothers who had recently been beating each other up in a storeroom.

When he released me, he did a grand sweeping gesture with his hand.

"We do yoga right here!" he said.

Oh, if only we could, I thought. And then I thought again: *Wait, what if this is yoga, or at least part of yoga?* But that thought seemed too sincere to me, so instead I said, "Nah, yoga's boring. Let's have a drink."

We were having trouble getting into a certain pose. Richard told us to practice by squatting, "like a king, not a peasant." He said: "When I first started doing yoga, I was very stiff, and all my poses looked the same. Then I went to India and I got hepatitis A and amoebic dysentery. I spent two weeks"—he squatted—"in this position. When I finally stood up, I'd lost a lot of weight, but also, because I'd been squatting, all the poses were easier for me."

Those of us in the west, he said, suffer from "the curse of the chair."

Well, I certainly experienced the curse of the chair. Compared with many of my fellow practitioners, with their nice yoga bodies and their 5:30 AM meditation practice by the pool, I felt like an aging water buffalo, incapable of doing much. My back had begun to hurt again, from where I'd pulled it during Bikram. By day four of our brutal *asana* practice, I couldn't bend forward at all. Richard noticed this, and he came over to inquire. I showed him the area. He nodded knowingly, raised one eyebrow, and said, "take your tiiiiiiime."

It was the best advice a yoga teacher had ever given to me, though maybe not that surprising coming from a guy who, earlier that day, had described yoga as "kung fu for hermits." I did, indeed, take my time, and didn't push myself too hard. As a result, the practice was perfect and transcendent.

"Blessed are the stiff," Richard said to us all. "The flexible are cursed. People are very disappointed when they get their chin to their shin. It's all still breath and the spaces in between. There's nothing else."

Afterward, I walked around on a cloud of bliss. My brain appeared to be functioning differently. While taking a whiz at the urinal, I gazed at an ant crawling up the wall, my mouth agape, with total wonder that a creature such as this could exist. I found myself staring at a palm tree and uttering an involuntary "hmm" of ecstatic curiosity. The sunlight glistening off someone's face seemed like a miracle. At breakfast, I closed my eyes and opened my ears to the multilingual chatter around me. It sounded like the world before the Tower of Babel collapsed, marvelous and unique.

Walking down the road to a convenience store so I could buy some crappy factory-made cookies, I saw a dead cat on the side of the road. This made me a bit sad. It seemed like the creature had died unfairly and cruelly. A few days later, walking past the same spot, I saw a cat skeleton, with just a little liquid *schmutz* around the body. The heat had made fast work of what had once been a cat body. But rather than think, "oh, man, that's gross," I instead gazed at the corpse with fascination. *All matter was constantly transforming,* I thought. *And that is the true nature of the universe.*

Mind you, I was sober at the moment I had this thought. What was happening to my mind? It only got worse during the afternoon *sutra* sessions. The first twenty minutes were relentlessly hilarious because Richard had begun teaching us Sanskrit consonants, and we chanted them along with the vowel sounds, leading to a roomful of adults singing, without irony, the following:

"Pa pa, pee pee, poo poo."

I convulsed, puffed out my cheeks, and did everything I could not to burst out laughing. Other than one mischievous Austrian guy named Helmut, who I'd been drinking with at the Easy Time, no one seemed to join me. Perhaps they thought I was practicing some sort of complicated *pranayama* move.

After that, out of Richard's mouth came an uninterrupted stream of learned wisdom. I can't really encompass the reality of what he said. I just sat there in wonder half the time, and, as such, took bad notes, ignoring a lot of the important stuff and writing down useless crap like:

"Using the mind, you create a scaffolding where free thought flows between the boundaries of the dialectic."

But, for the most part, I think I grasped his central message. Any yoga practice, he said, will eventually serve you up a "plate of rocks." Life will become difficult and you will suffer, and you have to stick with your practice through the crisis. We become over-attached to pleasant experience out of fear of suffering, he said, and that just creates more suffering because the pleasant experiences, like all experiences, must eventually end.

Facing impermanence, he said, is the hardest thing that a human being can do. We'd really rather not to think about it at all. But once you start to feel and understand impermanence, you get a "higher taste." You experience the unlimited delight of yoga. Nothing compares to the sense of freedom you get from accepting impermanence. It's difficult, yes, but the difficulty seems like nothing compared with what you get in return. That's when you want to teach, when you want to share. The ultimate challenge, he said, difficult for even the most advanced yogis, is to accept the fact that you're going to die, possibly soon, and to realize your own death as just another in a series of transformations illumined by the all-seeing light of pure awareness.

"Yoga is rehearsal for death," he said.

This chipper message seemed to directly contradict the "open your heart to the possibilities of the universe" school of yoga-chat, which so seemed to dominate discourse in my part of the world. I'd never bought into that stuff, but what Richard said resonated very strongly with me, even though he'd promised us nothing, other than disciplined attention to a new habit of mind.

I was sitting at a table, moving my steamed vegetables around with a fork as I thought about this. A nice woman from Singapore somehow managed to get my attention.

"I was practicing behind you today," she said. "What's wrong with your back?"

"Oh, I pulled a muscle a few months ago."

"No, I meant all those red dots."

"Those are zits."

"What are zits?"

"You know, pimples. Acne."

"You need some sun and salt water."

"I'll just keep my shirt on. It will reduce suffering."

"Oh, no, it gives me a good gazing point."

From then on, I practiced in the back row.

One afternoon, after we'd graduated from singing the Sanskrit alphabet, Richard said that we were going to do a certain chant five or six times. And then we were going to sit for five minutes. The residue from the chant would hang around, and then we'd see what happened.

So we chanted, and then we sat. It was the first time I'd ever meditated. I scooted my shoulder bag out of the way, propped myself up with a couple of cushions, and closed my eyes. At first, I was aware of a twinge in my knee. I noticed the twinge, and then it passed me by and it didn't hurt anymore. Then, there was an equivalent twinge in my back. This, too, I noticed and let go. After that, I went inside. Vague impressions, voices, thoughts, memories, ideas, and images flowed by in a continual stream, no one more important than the next, all equal, all different, none really mattering except for the moment of noticing them. My mind floated free, untethered and undisturbed.

At some point, I heard Richard say, "thank you," and then I returned. To what, I don't know. All I knew was that I'd felt tired when I started, and now I was no longer tired. Whatever had happened to me transcended rest.

Afterward, at dinner, I went up to Richard.

"That was my first meditation experience," I said.

"Really?" he said. "I'm glad to have been there."

"Yeah, thank you," I said. "It was really cool."

"Well," he said, "it certainly does bring on an altered state of consciousness."

Meditation was going to be easy!

The next day, we meditated again. It was obscenely hot outside, and I'd come to class straight from the pool at the Easy Time. I wore my bathing suit, and no shirt. This would have been fine, except that the suit was still wet, and all those attractive, equally near-naked bodies surrounded me, and, also I dripped with sweat. Sure enough, just as we began, I felt a stirring below.

Oh no, I thought. *I can't get a boner while meditating. That just wouldn't be appropriate.* But I did. A nice little chubby threatened to poke through the Velcro, as if to say, "I want to meditate, too." Clearly, it had to be stopped. I tried to notice the boner and move on, but it turns out that if you meditate on your boner, the boner just gets stronger. Or does it? Yes, I decided, it does, and did. I should have known, since I'd been meditating on my boner for nearly three decades. But it had never come up, not seriously anyway, in a yoga context before.

Well, at least no one was looking. Or were they? I couldn't tell, because I had my eyes closed. Still, the one-eyed snake yipped away in my swim trousers. I tried to think of non-boner things, like old ladies, or dead dogs, or Joe Biden, but that didn't work because if you meditate properly, thoughts leave your mind as soon as they end. So I was just going to have to accept my stiffy. Then I lost control of all conscious thought, and when Richard rang the bell fifteen minutes later, my boner had, mercifully, vanished. Truly, yoga was a wondrous thing.

After class, a student of Richard's, who'd been with him a long time, approached him as he put the finishing sips on that day's mango *lassi*.

"Richard," she said, "now that Patthabi Jois is gone, can people call you *guruji*?"

Guruji means most revered and highest master. Even though, in my mind, Richard qualified, he didn't pause in answering.

"No," he said. "No one can call me *guruji*."

Now he paused.

"Maybe they can call me *dude-ji*," he said.

I doubted that would happen. But no possible nickname could fit him better. My *dude-ji* had taught me so much. In fact, he'd taught me not to revere him as *dude-ji* at all. During one sutra talk, he said, "There's this myth of omniscience, where the yogi knows everything."

Ah, he said, but that's not the case at all. The danger of contemporary yoga is that lineages get broken down. Teachers pass on physical tricks, but they can't really pass down the feeling of "not me," of non-existence. Yoga, he said, is designed to humble you, to "trim the ego of the modalities of practice," or, more prosaically, to "drive you crazy."

"If you're lucky," he said, "the primary series gets you. The poses are designed to get harder and harder until one day, you realize the body doesn't matter, and you go, ohhhhhhhh. *Guruji* would give me yoga poses that I'm sure didn't even exist, because if you looked at them biomechanically, they weren't possible. And he'd say, "Ohhh. Very weak today.""

Nothing is cool, nothing is special, he said. Experience is everything, and what your ego does with the experience means nothing.

"But you *are* special," insisted one of the students.

"No I'm not," Richard said.

"But the Dalai Lama is special."

"No he's not. He's empty."

"But *guruji* was special."

"No he wasn't."

Later, I walked down the road back to Easy Time with another student, who'd been with Richard, on and off, for a long time.

"I really enjoyed that today," I said.

"Yeah," she said. "But really he's just empty. That's why he's such an effective teacher."

"Still, it's cool that he has so much knowledge."

"He wouldn't say that."

"Yeah, but I would."

"So many teachers," she said, "it's about their own ego. It's about creating a cult. They tell their students they're great, and their students tell them they're great, and it just perpetuates a cycle of misery. They're just creating *samskara*."

It's not like I disagreed with her, entirely, but she could have looked me in the eye when she said that. Shut the fuck up, you pompous Buddhist automaton, I wanted to say. But I didn't, because it just would have led to more suffering.

By the beginning of the second week, we'd all turned into yoga zombies, albeit vegetarian ones. We went about our business mechanically, perhaps going for a dip, and having the same conversations over and over: Who do you study with? Do you have a *pranayama* practice? How much are the massages at *your* hotel? I spent most of my time between sessions thinking about my next meal, and I even slept through a couple of morning practices, without worrying or caring. My brain and body had been flushed clean.

Mostly, I bobbed around in the pool at the Easy Time, with about a dozen other people, determined to live the good life between sessions where we either suffered or talked incessantly *about* suffering. At some point, we turned the corner and now the workshop moved toward its close. We talked about what we'd do after it ended.

"I think I'm going to start teaching," I said.

This stunned me even as it came out of my mouth. I hadn't really considered teaching, not seriously, especially because I wasn't certified. But Richard's blanket dismissal of certification had given me courage. However, a more veteran student of Richard's, and of the yogic arts in general, seemed skeptical. During the retreat, we dealt with each other warily, though we did later exchange some nice messages on Facebook.

"What do you want to teach?" she asked.

"I don't know," I said. "Maybe the *sutras*?"

"I'd be very careful before I did that."

"Why?"

"It's dangerous to spread the *dharma* before you've experienced some of the things it talks about."

First of all, how did she know I *hadn't* experienced some of those things? Second of all, who was she to tell me not to teach? Third, didn't Richard expressly disdain the idea of qualification? If I wanted to teach, I should teach. The fourth question, I spoke aloud.

"Um," I said. "What's the *dharma*?"

"The teachings," she said, sourly.

"Oh, right," I said.

"Seriously," she said. "You have to be careful. If you tell someone the wrong thing, you could ruin their life."

"OK," I said. "I'll keep that in mind."

"Good."

"So what are *you* doing after the retreat?" I asked.

"Oh, I'm going to Bali for a week," she said. "I'm a brat. I know it."

With that, she drifted away.

I briefly felt jealous that she was going to Bali after Thailand. But my yoga practice was strong at that point, so I managed to put it aside. Jealousy was a useless emotion, a *vrtti*, a poisonous distraction from the luminous true reality of pure awareness.

Instead, I realized, I'd just announced my intention to teach yoga. I felt like an unlikely candidate. Richard, had, in class, been talking about the concept of *bhoga*, which, in Sanskrit, means "material enjoyment." It also means "unoffered foodstuffs," but the first definition is somewhat more relevant to our purposes. In India, he said, it's an insult when people call you a "bhogi yogi." That means you're an unserious Westerner who's visiting the yoga motherland primarily to have a good time on the cheap. Indulging yourself heedlessly flies in the face of true yoga practice. In the *Bhagavad Gita*, Krishna tells Arjuna that he won't be able to fully practice yoga until he renounces all attachments to "sense objects." No more *bhoga* for you, dude.

On the other hand, Richard said, he once knew a macrobiotic guy in Chicago, and he took Richard to an ashram. They spent all day being very healthy. On a break, they went outside. In the alley, two guys were very happily sharing a huge tub of ice cream. "The happiest guys are always in the alley, smoking," said Dude-Ji.

At that moment, two different people turned around, looked at me, smiled, and said "Easy Time."

"You're right," Richard said. "Easy Time. But don't get attached."

That concept, I could teach.

One night I stuck around Yoga Thailand after not eating my dinner. The staff put on a video about life in Mysore. This featured archival footage, from some time in the '80s, of *guruji* leading his shala with a group of master students, including Richard. We all got a kick out of watching *guruji* slap his hands on a hot yogini's ass. Then he appeared to mount her like a stallion on mating day. Standards of propriety are, or at least were, different in India, I suppose. We also got to watch twenty-five-year-old footage of Dude-Ji getting a hot oil massage.

That was too strange for me, so it was back to Easy Time for fried dough balls. Every meal began with these, accompanied by a homemade tomato sauce, and ended with a round of *limoncello* shots, compliments of the house. Maybe I *was* a *bhogi* yogi. So I wanted to have a good time. So what? This was a hell of a long way to travel to have a bad time.

An Easy Time coalition of sorts had formed. We considered ourselves the fun ones who knew how to live properly. Of course, this was totally obnoxious, judgmental, and non-yogic, not to mention untrue. In the evenings, we drank wine and beer and ate pizza, sometimes even Thai food. We played baccarat, betting a round of drinks or a round of Easy Time's fantastic homemade *tiramisu*.

Toward the end of the second week, our little group determined that Dude-Ji should join us for dinner at the Easy Time. This would be the crowning night of his experience in Thailand, we said. He'd be the honored guest at the ultimate Easy Time dinner party. We began to whisper absurd plans. Helmut, my Austrian friend, took charge along with his Romanian wife Gloria, a former mortician. Together, they owned two businesses: one selling weapons to the local police, and the other, newsprint to the local papers, meaning their livelihoods more or less depended on an uptick in organized crime. Fortunately for them, they lived in Bucharest, where organized crime is always upticking, and therefore were able to afford a yoga vacation in Thailand.

We gathered by the pool, trying to pull together a guest list. We'd decided on eight as the perfect number. Anything else could become unruly. There were several qualifications for dinner with Dude-Ji. The first, intelligence, eliminated virtually no one, since Ashtanga attracts a fairly intellectual crowd. The second, reasonable physical attractiveness, also didn't help narrow the field. We also looked for the right mix of funny and serious, young and middle-aged, cheery, and bitter. The final, deciding, intangibly quality, though, was totally arbitrary. Were they able to have an Easy Time? To our minds, any transgression from the ascetic norms of Yoga Thailand, however minor, merited consideration for our grand feast.

Our conversations went like this:

"What about so-and-so?" I would say.

"He eat the calzone," said Gloria.

"And he drink the wine," said Helmut.

"He in," said I.

Thursday evening arrived. Helmut and Gloria had skipped class because of some sort of business emergency back in Bucharest, so the job of escorting Richard to the Easy Time was left to me and yet *another* Austrian, Maria, who'd been my best friend throughout the conference. We both had the social skills necessary to get Dude-Ji fifty meters down the road.

After *sutra* class, I informed Richard that I'd be his guide. He looked up at me.

"Oh," he said, as though I'd just taken shape in front of him, like a teleporting Starfleet member. He did this a lot. Life, to him, was a series of discrete occurrences, and he viewed each one with a fresh eye.

Richard, Maria, and I began to amble down the road together. Suddenly she stopped and put her hands on her hips.

"You are *not* going to wear that to dinner," she said.

He was wearing his usual yoga uniform: tank top and shorts.

"But it's hot and I'm comfortable," he said.

Maria looked at him sternly. She'd just come from two years of managing a Chinese art gallery in Shanghai, where she'd regularly dealt with tougher customers than *this* aging hippie. She may have respected Dude-Ji, but she wasn't going to let him get away with slovenliness.

Richard cleared his throat.

"I'm just going to go back to my room and put away my bag," he said.

Maria and I made patterns in the dirt with our feet for about five minutes. The sun was setting, yet still we dripped with sweat. The air smelled like sea salt and rotting durian. Then Richard came striding happily down the road, beaming like a boy getting his class photo taken. He wore a Hawaiian shirt with hints of pink and blue scattered throughout. It had faded quite a bit since he'd bought it in the early 1990s. But it did have a collar. *Now* he was dressed properly for dinner.

Helmut and Gloria had dealt with their crisis and secured the table. Together, we'd set dinner conversation rules. Under no circumstances were we to talk about yoga *unless* Richard brought it up. This seemed to work very well. The conversation flowed, especially once the house started pouring one of the three bottles of wine for the table. Richard said he wanted just a "taste" of wine. His taste ended up being an entire glass, though he did refuse a refill.

Tongues loosened. Maria and I got into a heated argument about whether or not Cambodians were happier than Westerners because their lives were "simpler" than ours. She accused me of cynicism and inexperience, since she'd actually *been* to Cambodia. I accused her of *noblesse oblige* and quoted the lyrics to *Holiday in Cambodia*, of which no one had ever heard. This made me feel simultaneously old and American. Richard didn't really help matters, because he said he agreed with both of us.

Food arrived. Richard got a nice-looking Mediterranean salad. He took a bit and a look of pure refreshment spread over his face.

"That's why I liked living in Iran," he said. "The food all looked and tasted like this, as opposed to India, where everything is heavy and fried."

"Wait," I said. "When'd you live in Iran?"

"Oh, in the '70s," he said. He'd gone over there to study Sufi mysticism and had ended up teaching yoga to the Shah's children. It had really been quite an interesting experience. The Iranians were a very sophisticated and passionate people, Richard said. Around 1978, people started throwing rocks at him in public, and he knew it was time to leave.

We all gazed at him open-mouthed. How did this guy expect us to think that he wasn't special? From there, the conversation skidded a bit, and kept going only because Helmut had drunk about eight glasses of wine, which gave him the courage to babble on at great length about how practicing yoga had led him to understand his parents better. This gave the rest of us ammunition, and we enjoyed many happy minutes making fun of him.

Finally, the mighty *limoncello* shots arrived, compliments of the Easy Time.

Richard said, "Well, I only drink on special occasions . . ."

He looked around the table, grinned, and raised his glass.

After two weeks, we reached the end of the *sutras,* though we skipped most of Chapter 3, "The Extraordinary Powers," which makes all kinds of dangerous claims, for instance, that fully realized yogis can walk on water, eat glass, and such. These extraordinary powers are purported to exist:

In a biography, T. K. V. Desikchar writes that he once witnessed his father, the great Krishnamacharya, stop his heart and breath for six minutes, and then gradually return himself to life. When Desikachar asked his father to teach him, Krishnamacharya begged him not to ask again. That kind of knowledge, in the wrong hands, could be used for evil, he said, and to know how to do it is a curse. With extraordinary powers comes extraordinary responsibility. On a cheesier, more modern note, Bikram Choudhury once appeared on *That's Incredible* sandwiched between two beds of nails while his guru drove a motorcycle over him. Now that's non-attachment.

Richard kept it much simpler than that as we cruised to the close of Chapter 4. Ordinary powers would be just fine. Before we meditated, he said, "Out of twenty-five minutes, even if you only have one second where the mind cuts through, it's totally worth it." Then we arrived at *sutra* 29: "One who regards even the most exalted states disinterestedly, discriminating continuously between pure awareness and the phenomenal world, enters the final stage of integration, in which nature is seen to be a cloud of irreducible experiential substances."

At last, we'd arrived at *dharma-megha samadi*, the ultimate goal of all yoga. Had I finished? Was my yoga journey finally done?

No, Richard said. "You have to re-create and re-understand the *sutras* constantly. Even when you reach the highest state, you have to practice continually." For the past two weeks, Richard had been saying that "yoga ruins your life." I was beginning to understand what he meant. It was a lot of fucking work.

"The best thing," he said, "is to quit while you're ahead." We were ahead now, he said, so "any benefit that you've derived, let's dedicate it to other beings. Because all beings just want to be happy."

Then we chanted, and then we sat in bliss for a few seconds, but not much time passed before a Yoga Thailand staff member broke the silence by saying, "OK, is anyone here staying for next week's detox program?" Just like that, the spell had been snapped.

That clumsy end to such a magnificent experience left me depressed. Afterward, nothing awaited me but another buffet of limp, uninspired vegetables. I guess I expected a party on the last night, but everyone seemed even more subdued than usual. It would have been nice spending a few hours clinking beer bottles in the hot tub while singing "OLE, OLE OLE OLE!" or some other sort of Euro tackiness. Clearly, though, I was in the minority on that desire.

They served us "dessert" in the form of a plate of dry, flavorless cookies.

"Jesus fucking Christ," I said. "We paid them enough money. They could at least give us a proper cookie."

Helmut approached me, raising an eyebrow.

"You could put something on top of them . . ." he said.

He waved a cookie in front of my face. Atop it was a little brown nugget. It looked like a rat turd. Then I thought it might be a piece of smuggled European chocolate. Then I caught a whiff, and I suddenly realized his plan.

"Put that away!" someone shrieked. "Put it away!"

Yoga-Thailand, explicitly alcohol-free, probably wouldn't appreciate a hash-ball making its way around the *satsang*. So

I put it away the only way I knew how—into my mouth. I'd be seeing a cloud of irreducible experiential substances soon enough.

Then the scene shifted, and somehow I was walking by the front the desk of the Easy Time. The Rasta brother sat checking his email. He motioned me over.

"Hey, Mr. Neal," he said.

"Yes?" I said.

"You're from Los Angeles."

"Yes."

"I went to California once," he said. "Tijuana was fun."

Tijuana, I wanted to tell him, was in Mexico, but perhaps he already knew that. Also, I wanted to get the image of this guy attending a donkey show out of my head immediately. Because you know he did.

"You like Charles Bukowski?" he said.

In my stupor, I somehow believed that he said, "*Are* you like Charles Bukowski?"

"Well, I'm really nothing like Charles Bukowski," I said. "I'm a lot yuppier than he was, and, you know, way more neurotic . . ."

"*I* like Charles Bukowski," he said. "He's my favorite writer."

Oh, right, this guy had no idea that I was a writer. He just wanted to talk about Bukowski.

"Yeah," I said. "He's pretty damn cool."

I went to join my friends at our nightly drunken pizza gorge, already in progress. Soon, my head felt like it had blown up to the size of a balloon.

"Yoga is annoying!" I said. "Doesn't everyone think so?"

No one seemed to think so. Across the table, Helmut raised his eyebrows at me.

"How are you feeeeeeling?" he said.

"Same as you," I said.

"I don't thiiiiiink so . . ."

"You didn't eat any?"

"Nooooooo . . ."

"You bastard."

Later, Helmut, Gloria, and I took a stroll around the garden, looking at the moon. I realized that I'd horned in on their little date, but by the time we'd gone halfway around the pool, it was too late to bail. The hotel's owner staggered toward us.

"He doesn't look so good," Helmut said.

The Rastaman walked past, tripped over a bush, smacked his face into a coconut palm, bounced off, and then disappeared mumbling into the dark. I went upstairs, washed my face, got into bed, and opened my notebook. My head hit the pages immediately, and I began to drool. I fell asleep with my cheek resting on the book. When my alarm went off seven hours later, it had stained my face with ink. If a scuzzed-out Faye Dunaway had only been lying next to me, my Bukowskization would have been complete.

Then it was back to Yoga Thailand. Richard led us through a short, lovely, simple asana practice. I grabbed a quick breakfast and said a bunch of unsentimental good-byes. I'd deliberately booked my flight so I wouldn't have to linger.

Dude-Ji sat by himself at a table next to the juice bar. I went over to him and bowed.

"Thank you, sensei," I said.

"Oh, hey," he said, standing to shake my hand. "It was really fun having you."

"You gave me a lot of thoughts to observe," I said.

He laughed at my lame joke and said, "See you around."

"Probably," I said. "Take it easy."

With that, I felt complete. Since childhood, I'd struggled with myself, both conceptually and quite concretely; my soul had resonated with melodramatic pain. More than once, I had wandered out on an icy Chicago fishing pier and screamed "WHY?????" into the indifferent Lake Michigan night. These moments reoccurred, periodically, every couple of years. My yoga experiences had begun with a similar shattering. I now realized that my search for a "best self" had been off-kilter, or at least off message; I began to understand, or at least to suspect, that my self as I constructed it in my head didn't exist at all. In the face of the infinite and undefinable, how could anything that I'd ever done, said, thought, or felt possibly have any significance? It couldn't, because there was no "I." Therefore, with a clear mind and an open heart, I approached the front desk at Yoga Thailand.

"Good morning," I said. "I'd like to dispute a charge."

16

Ill (Not in a Good Way)

Swami Satchidananda, the founder of Integral Yoga, spoke at Woodstock in 1969, leading a chant and saying, "So, let all our actions, and all our arts, express yoga. Through the sacred art of music, let us find peace." Well, we all know how that worked out, but yoga persevered in the West nevertheless. In the summer of 2009, when the dull echoes of prefabricated nostalgia brought Woodstock, for the millionth time, back into the public consciousness, yoga actually turned the tables and did something new with the myth. This was the summer of the Wanderlust Festival, quite possibly the game-changing event in American yoga culture. *Bhoga* had triumphed.

Wanderlust sprang from the very Gen-X creative-class career paths of Jeff Krasno and Schuyler Grant, Columbia graduates and Williamsburg, Brooklyn, parents in their late thirties. He ran rock festivals, and she ran a yoga studio and high-end yoga retreats. At some point, they decided to combine the two, with the stipulation that yoga and rock 'n' roll receive equal billing. For the first time, yoga and music would be equivalent cultural forces. Two great upper-middle-class hobbies were about to merge under the high mountain sun.

The festival would take place in Squaw Valley, a ski resort that hovers above Lake Tahoe on the California side of the Sierras. The lodges and conference rooms would become yoga studios, and the ski lifts would take people to the top of the mountain, where they'd do yoga poolside and enjoy a lineup of musical acts that included Spoon, Andrew Bird, Gillian Welch, and the patron-saint of rock 'n' roll yoga culture, Michael Franti. Also, as always, MC Yogi would be dropping in for a few sets. If anything, the yoga programming was even more impressive. As headliners, they booked Shiva Rea, the queen of Trance Dance, and John Friend, the founder of *anusara* yoga. Along with Michael Franti and Spoon, they shared the biggest typefaces on the poster.

About six weeks before Wanderlust hit, I began to receive Facebook messages with links to the website. People wrote stuff like, "I saw this and it seemed like your gig." Why? Just because it was founded by yoga-freak Gen-X hipster parents? Well, OK, I could see how people could make the connection. But my interest was barely piqued.

I'd done a lot hard work trying to figure out what yoga meant to me, and I'd gathered some quiet, private lessons about suffering and the true nature of reality. For the first time in decades, my mind felt pretty clear. The last thing I needed was another distractingly weird yoga carnival. At the same time, a rock festival in Squaw Valley, with some yoga thrown in, sounded pretty cool. This could be a groundbreaking moment in the history of yoga culture. I'd be a holy fool to miss it. Oh, what to do?

Yoga Journal made the decision for me. About a week-and-a-half before the opening *asana*, they assigned me to write a piece about yoga festivals. As part of the piece, they insisted that I go to Wanderlust so I could convey a sense of the magical vibe.

So that's how, on a Friday morning, I found myself guiding my car (rented at the Reno airport) into the VIP parking garage at the Squaw Valley Resort. It would remain there, undriven, for forty-eight hours while I strolled light-headedly through a scene of unparalleled good feeling, wearing an extremely sexy ensemble of yoga shorts, sleeve-less shirts, hiking boots without socks, and an old, sweaty Dodgers cap. I felt like the festival's weird, smelly second cousin.

Within fifteen minutes of my arrival, I found myself atop the same garage where my car was parked, underneath a white tent, laying my mat down on some rental parquet floor. The occasion: a class given by Duncan Wong, creator of the trademarked Yogic Arts sequence. This is kind of an elegant form of yoga kung-fu, and Wong is kind of the Bruce Lee of yoga culture, compact and tattooed and sexu-ally charged.

"Did you study your sequence?" he asked us.

Most people nodded, but I, and a few others, said, "What sequence?"

An assistant passed out a laminated card, which featured Wong doing the sequence. I had never seen at least half the poses. A certain discomfort began to set in; then Wong introduced his assistant teacher, a lovely young woman. "You probably saw her on the cover of *Yoga Journal*," he said, to much applause.

Then we started to go through the poses slowly. Wong kept telling his DJ to turn the music up, then turn it down, and then up again. He touted his accomplishments as a pose-creator, fiddled with his mic headset, and made jokes like, "a man's mantra should be 'yes, dear, whatever you say dear.'" Also, he said that a subtle touch from a master yoga teacher can transform your practice and change you as a person.

"So if I touch your boob, it's no accident," he said.

The guy had definitely created a vigorous, beautiful flow sequence. He could probably snap me like a twig with a glance, if he so desired. Regardless, I wasn't buying. I quietly rolled up my mat and walked away.

"Good bye, so long, see you later," he said.

A report on a yoga blog later said: "Duncan Wong was pretty cool. He blasted Justin Timberlake. Then, in Warrior 1 pose, he turned on the hip hop super loud and told everyone to dance. We just broke out."

That's a long way, I thought, from *dude-ji* telling us to free our minds by accepting the reality of our impermanence. In fact, the overarching feeling at Wanderlust was: We're youngish and fit and happy and we're going to live forever! *Lies*, I thought. *All lies.*

I took a gondola up to the top of the mountain, to see what I could see. I saw another mountain, and also a crystal lake and a valley at once mystically rocky and verdant. They'd had a lot of rain at Squaw recently, and it showed. As we approached the top, I bore witness to a staggeringly hot woman in a red bikini. She lay atop the outcropped rock wall of a lookout point, and then, in full view of the gondola, pushed up into a flawless wheel pose. A man took her picture while she did this.

"Look, honey," said a grandma tourist to a kid tourist. "She's doing her yoga."

But was she? Wasn't yoga supposed to be something private, quiet, and sacred? This chick looked like she was posing for the *Sports Illustrated* yoga issue. She *knew* she looked good. When we got to the top, I saw her taking a picture of the guy, who was just as hot. He'd removed his shirt, and was currently displaying his magnificent side-plank to the Valley, Tahoe, and beyond. The woman now wore a crushed-straw cowboy hat, a *de rigeur* Wanderlust accessory. The ego parade continued.

You assholes, I thought to myself. *You're going to die, too, you know.*

Anyone who thinks of yoga as high-priced self-empowerment for the over-privileged creative class would have found a lot of evidence to affirm their thesis that weekend in Squaw Valley. Half of the Bay Area had made the drive across California, and they were celebrating in groovy, self-righteous togetherness. But something else was also occurring. At Bonarroo, Coachella, or the Austin City Limits Festival, all of which sprang from the same company that planned Wanderlust, the music-festival experience was about grinding down, exhausting, tapping all party resources until you suffered a massive sonic hangover. Though I tried mightily, it was hard to feel like shit for long at Wanderlust.

Before I left town, I'd spoken to Schuyler Grant, the yoga teacher who'd served as the inspiration for the whole kaboodle. She said, "Like most modern practitioners, we're not ascetic. We have our yoga lives, and then we go off and have a beer or whatever. It's so fractured. But how great to attend one event and have both. How great to dance until 2 AM, have exactly what you have in a long music event, but, at the same time, feel really good?"

Then she offered to have her mother babysit Elijah, for free, so I could bring my wife up to Squaw Valley with me next time. You just can't stay annoyed at yoga people. They're all so freaking *nice*.

Soon, I found myself under the calming spell of Doug Swenson, vegan, surfer, and former Tahoe City health food store owner. Swenson told us that he'd grown up in Texas in the 1960s, where you had to keep your yoga a secret if you wanted to stay alive. He ended up teaching his younger brother, David, who actually became the better known of the Swenson brothers. But both guys evolved into Ashtanga masters. Doug had a laid-back, funny style. We did an easy, end-of-the-week practice. He didn't promise universal happiness or claim copyrights on his poses. I vowed to follow him for the rest of the weekend.

That night, the "Kula Village" at the bottom of the mountain had a mild Burning Man vibe going. People wearing bird headdresses walked around on stilts. Young snarky clowns strolled arm-in-arm while smoking cigarettes. Onstage, an art-rock ensemble called The Mutaytors put on an impressive display of face-painted fire dancing, which created quite a frenzy in the audience. After they finished, I had the immense privilege of seeing Sharon Jones and the Dap Kings for the first time. Jones was 4 feet 11 inches of roiling neo-soul energy, and the crowd ate her for a snack. She decided she needed a man to come up on stage to give her some lovin'. A skinny kid rose out of the crowd and took the stage. Jones rubbed against him. He seemed receptive.

"Oh my God!" someone shouted. "She's got a gay little yoga boy!"

Now we were having fun. On the way back to my room, I bought a four-dollar "organic melon salad" from a guy selling them off a card table. It looked delicious and fresh, and was a real bargain in the land of the twelve-buck smoothie. A good deal, a great band, and some relaxing yoga sent me to bed in a damn fine mood. I went to sleep expecting more of the same the following day.

This was the wrong thought. The *sutras* teach that attachment leads to suffering. I'd become overly attached to pleasure. Where do you think that led?

I awoke early with the intention of going to a Doug Swenson class called Ashtanga with Extra Spice. My head hurt so much, though, that a simple forward bend might have caused it to explode. Nevertheless, I went in search of the extra spice, but it had been moved to a different conference center across the compound. Walking a quarter-mile, very fast, seemed impossible just then.

Though I just wanted to lie down in the dirt and die, I can say for certain that I didn't have a hangover. The night before, I'd consumed one beer and two pulls off a stranger's weed pipe. Some days, I had that much before breakfast. It certainly wasn't enough to knock me on my ass. No, this was something else, a weird hybrid of altitude sickness, dehydration, and yoga *weltschmerz*. *Perhaps I'd best take it easy,* I thought.

The best course would involve meditation. I went to a 9 AM *vipassana* class, led by a guy named Wes from the venerable Spirit Rock Center, in Marin County, California. According to the Spirit Rock website, *vipassana,* or "insight" meditation "is a simple technique which has been practiced in Asia for over twenty-five hundred years. Beginning with the focusing of attention on the breath, the practice concentrates and calms the mind. It allows one to see through the mind's conditioning and thereby to live more fully present in the moment."

Despite the fact that Wes looked a lot like Joe Pesci, he had much calm wisdom to impart. He led us through a couple of short but lovely meditations, saying that one really needed to go on a meditation retreat to get the full benefit. I saw the present moment all too clearly.

Oh, please don't let me barf, I thought. *I'm tired of barfing on yoga vacations.* But my headache had begun traveling throughout my entire body. The great purge was near.

I meditated on this for an hour, and then busted ass back to my room, flinging open the door, running to the bathroom, and barely arriving in time to unleash a torrent of half-digested organic melon salad into the bowl. Moaning audaciously, I repeated the pose three times. *Maybe I should copyright it,* I thought. It seemed to be my signature. I could call it downward-facing yack.

That would be the only *asana* I'd do for the rest of the weekend. I'd learned my lesson too well in Thailand, and knew that if I dared try another class, I'd find myself vomiting in a public bathroom, with no staff nurse to come to my aid. Fortunately, I had several fizzy electrolyte tabs in my swag bag. I ate three tabs, each accompanied by a stainless steel Swedish bottleful of water. By the time I'd drunk my third bottle, I felt as bloated as an elephant seal, but I wasn't going to barf again.

For the rest of the day, I wandered through a wide world of *vritti*: a seemingly endless outdoor "Eco Village" boutique of yoga wear, gear, retreats, schools, and the occasional non-profit cause, outdoor equipment gear demonstration, food and drink booths from environmentally friendly companies like Honest Tea and Anheuser-Busch, a "Geodome" art house sponsored by Converse, and the Play Lounge, "a magical outdoor adult play space filled with opportunities to explore freedom, expression, connection, and the joyful child within." These included Silk Sanctuary, Bohemian Bar, Love Bag, and, of course, Hoop Dance. I saw people messing around on tightropes and pommel horses and relaxing in comfy pillows. It was all completely absurd. Both up the mountain and down, the ladies of San Francisco were spinning hoops around their perfectly formed yoga hips. After a while, I just wanted to toss all those goddamn hoops into the lake.

I took the gondola to the top of the mountain for one of the festival's signature events, a class with John Friend, the founder of *anusara* yoga. Friend is a curly haired teddy bear of a man who just exudes good humor and happiness. The archetypal image of the festival, which appeared in the

New York Times, shows him, chest shot forward and arms up to the sky, leading more than one hundred sunglass-and-headband wearing people through glorious yoga bliss at more than eight thousand feet. It was all bourgeois sun, fun, and joy, and I was there.

Upon a splintery wooden deck overlooking all of Squaw Valley and Lake Tahoe, Friend encouraged everyone to "touch the sky and soften to the magnificence of where we are." I stood and watched as everyone chanted; their faces glistened with bliss. Friend told them about the "first principle" of yoga: "Take it eaaaaasy," he said. "Relax. Enjoy. Chill out. Melt your heart and open to something bigger." This stood in direct contrast to the "first principle" that *dude-ji* had taught us in Thailand, that everything was impermanent and therefore creates suffering. Friend's pill was a lot easier to swallow. No wonder *anusara* is so popular.

After a while, I grew bored of watching one hundred people (including Duncan Wong, who was wearing a purple-and-white striped Speedo) enjoying themselves to the max. I don't really love practicing ass-to-nose at eight thousand feet while a half-dozen photographers move through the crowd. For me, at least, that defeats the purpose. So I went and sat in the hot tub for a couple of hours.

From there, I wandered over to the Gold Coast stage, where the rock had been going since noon. There was a crowd, but it probably numbered about a third of what an outdoor venue like, say, Ravinia in Chicago draws on a Friday night. Wanderlust sold a ton of yoga tickets. The indie-rock people mostly stayed home. Yoga had moved to first position. Guitarist and singer Kaki King mounted a faint yowl of protest in the *Times* when she said, "I'm not going to do the hippie dance. I'm going to put shoes on and I'm not going to drink any mold . . . I'm not going to do any yoga."

Here, though, she numbered in the vast minority. I took a ski lift back down to the bottom. From one thousand feet above, it looked like hundreds of people were sitting on blankets near the foot of the lift, maybe having a picnic, watching music on a stage. Suddenly, every one of those people pushed up, as one, into downward dog. From my vantage, it looked like the earth had actually moved.

At the bottom, Shiva Rea was holding court on the same stage that Sharon Jones had dominated the night before. Wanderlust had advertised this as the world's biggest yoga class, eight hundred people strong, because she was supposed to be backed by Michael Franti. But two days before the festival, Franti was diagnosed with a ruptured appendix. There'd be no Wanderlust for him.

Instead, The Mutaytors backed up Shiva Rea and did a very nice job. I counted two hundred and fifty students, maximum. People practiced in the full sun, under the shade of pine trees, and I saw more than one person doing *vinyasa* in the dirt, without a mat.

Shiva Rea asked the crowd, "How many of you are teachers?" At least half raised their hands. "Then you're river guides," she said.

From there, it was back up the mountain to see Gillian Welch and David Rawlings play bluegrass like it was meant to be played. It had been years I'd seen them last, and they'd gotten even better. "I think this is the first time I've ever gotten to a gig in a gondola," Welch said. Meanwhile, over by the lift, the Wanderlust people had put up a get-well poster to Michael Franti for everyone to autograph, along with a sign that read: "Michael Franti is ill (not in a good way)."

The evening progressed and I found myself in a hotel room with four barely interested people, trying to explain the *suara*, the little dot accent that you see written over the *m* in the Sanskrit transliteration of OM.

"It can't come from your lips," I explained. "It has to come from your soft palate and the sound needs to travel up into your head like an endless snake."

We'd been smoking weed out of a beer-can bong, and I was in a similar frame of mind when I went to see a 10:30 PM appearance by Girl Talk, the stage name of a Pittsburgh-based mash-up artist named Gregg Gillis. It's amazing that one guy with two laptops can whirl the crowd into such a frenzy, but there we were, in the audience, screaming with recognition at Girl Talk's clever mixes. From the stage, hot chicks in dominatrix costumes continually unspooled rolls of toilet paper over our heads, using some sort of gun-like device.

"These are audiences with open minds," Gillis later told the *Times*. "Even if they're not into it, they're not there to critique it. And if they like it, they're not embarrassed to get into it."

I felt hands on my shoulders. A woman, who I'd never seen before and never would again, spun me around and gave me a kiss on the cheek. Then she went back to grinding against her boyfriend.

"Man," she said. "Sometimes you know you've ended up in the right place."

At that moment, I had to agree.

17

Club Sutra

I received an email from Mara. It read: "Wanna open a yoga studio in Eagle Rock with me?" It was an attractive idea. At last, I'd have a "third place" that could serve as my unofficial home in Los Angeles, where my friends could hang out and bask in my newfound yogic glow. I approached Regina with the idea.

"No way," she said.

"Why not?"

"Because you're not a yoga teacher."

"Not yet."

"Goddammit, Pollack, you always do this. You thought you were a rock star, but you weren't. You thought you were a cool dad, and you weren't."

"Wait a second, I *am* a cool dad."

"You know what I mean."

I did. Yet the idea didn't lose its appeal. On Fridays, after class, Mara started asking me out for coffee. She really wanted to open this studio. I said I'd be an "advice guy." Maybe I could hook her up with some investors, and I could certainly help with publicity. I uttered a lot of sentences that started with, "What you need to do is . . ."

Finally, she said, "Stop telling me what I need to do. I need to hear 'we.'"

The thought of using Quicken or an Excel spreadsheet, she said, terrified her. "We'd have to rent a credit-card machine," she added. "So are you in or out?"

I thought. I don't want to be financially liable for a yoga studio. The operating costs would be substantial. There'd be rent. We'd have to buy equipment and pay the instructors. Most likely, there'd be a build-out. I wanted nothing to do with any of that. *I have a career already,* I thought. I don't need this, at all.

"I'm in," I said.

Mara scheduled our first business meeting. It would be held at the home of Linda Richards, otherwise known as Prabhu Prakash. Linda had a lot of business experience and had flirted in the past with the idea of opening a yoga studio herself. We drove over together, in Mara's car. I blathered on about how our yoga studio needed to be totally rock 'n' roll. It had to have an "indie aesthetic." We parked. I opened the door. A hot pain seized the right side of my lower back, and I tumbled out onto the sidewalk.

"ARRRRRGH!" I said.

"Neal," Mara said. "Did you just fall out of my car?"

"Yes!" I said. "I'm almost forty years old!"

After spending a couple of minutes on my hands and knees, I somehow made it to Linda's front door, with Mara propping me up. Within a minute, I was lying on a sheepskin rug, my legs at a ninety-degree angle. While I stayed prone, Linda made some homemade carrot-apple-ginger-beet juice. We ate tabbouleh salad, and started doing the numbers. I propped myself up.

"What we're looking to do is . . . ARRRRGH!"

My back had seized again. So for the rest of the meeting, I stared at the ceiling. The conversation seemed hazy. It felt like someone was running a Garden Weasel across my lumbar spine. Mara continued to have her strange aversion to "studio software." She insisted that she wanted to keep track of students on index cards. Linda and I had to keep reminding her that it wasn't 1975 anymore. Students expected a little more than that. In any case, the numbers worked out fine, assuming we could find someone to give us $75,000. At that moment, for me at least, I just wanted someone to give me two Demerol.

At some point, probably when I stood up and saw that my torso had shifted to the left, completely away from my hips, I realized that I wasn't going to be able to drive. Standing up required supreme effort. Mara somehow got me back to her house, but I wasn't going any further.

Regina arrived. When she saw me, she said, "Yeah, that's just what you looked liked after Bikram." She decided to take me to the doctor, but as we were walking across the street to the car, my back locked up, and I howled.

"That's it," she said. "We're going to the emergency room."

"Just get me to the fucking car," I said.

Two hours later, with our kid in tow, I staggered into my doctor's office. Within minutes, I was on my stomach, getting moist heat applied to the damaged area. The chiropractor entered. He placed hands, and then pulled back.

"Whoa," he said. "This is gonna be tough."

"What?" I said.

"Your muscles are frozen."

"Great."

He explored along my low mid-back, and I heard a pop. That particular joint along the spine, he said, had been out of place, and it had led to the straining of a lower-back muscle.

"Is that it?" I said. "A strained muscle?"

"Yep."

I attempted to push myself up to a sitting position. About halfway, my strained muscle tightened. It felt like someone was ripping my back open with a claw.

"AAAAAAAAAAAH!" I said, and then I took the name of someone else's Lord in vain.

Lately, at Mara's, I'd been trying to bend backwards into wheel pose from a standing position. I vowed to cut that out of my practice. First, though, I had to get off the chiropractor's table. The doctor had me roll onto my side and dangle my feet off the table for ballast. I got halfway up before my back seized again, and I collapsed onto the table with a scream. Then we tried the other side, with the same result, and then again, with the tight, stabbing pain accompanied by a guttural howl of agony. Clearly, I needed more treatment.

He hooked me up to a machine that emitted electrical impulses. This was a "nerve blocker," he said. He tested out various settings, and told me to find one where I didn't feel anything. So I did, and then I looked up.

"That's the weakest possible setting," he said. "*That's* how tight your muscles are."

When I stopped feeling sensation, he said, I needed to raise the levels very slightly. Any more than that, and I'd go through the roof. Since I'd be there a while, I asked him to send in the family.

"How's it going, baby?" Regina asked.

"Well, I'm hooked up to this machine that's sending electrical impulses to my muscles so I can fool my body into letting me get off the table."

"Oh."

"How's it going with you?"

"We're looking at magazines, and Elijah is running up and down the corridor."

"Mommy," Elijah said, "Show him the picture of the cat who has to go to the bathroom."

Eventually, my wife and son decided it was more fun to look at Lolcats than to watch me writhe in pain. The doctor returned, and we tried again. Neither side appeared to have improved.

"I'm never getting out of here," I said.

"Oh, yes you are," he said.

Next, we tried sliding me off the end of the table, onto my knees. He told me to curl my toes so my legs could get used to bearing weight again. I moved back and forth on my toes, getting a little more weight each time. I tried standing, but the pain was far worse than before. I grasped for the table, trying to pull myself to comfort.

The doctor put a rubber cover on his thumb to protect me from bruising and smacked my abs, trying to get a counter-reaction from my back. He went over me with a weird multi-pronged massage ball. I tried to stand again, didn't get there, and missed the table on the way down.

Now I was lying on the floor.

I pushed up into cobra position, and then onto my hands and knees. This required tremendous effort, and I stayed there, heaving and sweaty, feeling completely wrung out and looking like James Naughton mid-transformation in *An American Werewolf in London*.

"Man," said the chiropractor. "It makes me tired just watching you."

At this point, Regina and Elijah entered.

"Oh boy," Regina said.

"Maybe you should take him to the Chinese restaurant downstairs," I said.

"YAY!" said Elijah.

At least someone was happy. After they left, I realized I was feeling dizzy. The doctor got a caramel and popped it in my mouth while I was on my hands and knees. There were more attempts to stand, and more collapses to the floor. He got a paper cup of water, and then fizzed it with a magnesium tablet. Apparently, magnesium is a muscle relaxer. Since I couldn't sit up, I just raised my head slightly. He gave me little sips. Then I tried to stand up again, and collapsed again, screaming. By now, I'd been trapped in that little examining room for two-and-a-half hours.

If it wasn't for all my yoga, he said, I'd be exhausted by now, and unable to move. "I had a three-hundred-pound patient once," he added, "and it took him four hours to get off the floor."

That was enough. I couldn't lose, time-wise, to a three-hundred-pound man. I was in shape. I was a *yogi*. The sutras say that, "by mastering the flow of energy in the head and neck, one can walk through water, mud, thorns, and other obstacles without touching down, but rather floating over them." I thought of that, and I also thought of that scene in *All the Pretty Horses* where the main character cauterizes a suppurating wound by himself with a hot knife and nothing to dull the pain. I could do this!

I grabbed the table, lurched up, stuck my legs out behind me, and, very gradually, straightened my back.

"Just two percent more, and you're there," said the doctor.

I wrenched myself upward and gave a horrific yowl. No one heard it. My family was downstairs eating dumplings, and the office was empty except for a janitor. But once again, I stood erect.

"Wow, that must have hurt," the doctor said.

"It did."

"They never told me in medical school that I'd be staying until 8:30 at night trying to get a guy off the floor."

"Yeah, well," I replied, "they never told me in journalism school that I'd be trying to *get* off the floor at 8:30 at night."

"Good point," he said.

I spent the next fifteen minutes learning how to walk again, lurching around like Peter Boyle's character in *Young*

Frankenstein. At some point, I'd made sufficient progress for the doctor to go downstairs and get the car keys from Regina. Soon, he was walking me to the elevator, reminding me to take some Milk of Magnesia to loosen my stool, which would reduce pressure on the strained muscle.

I spent the next two days in bed, which gave me a lot of time to think. Obviously this was a sign telling me that under no circumstances should I ever consider becoming a partner in a yoga studio. Whatever sanity I'd built while doing yoga would quickly melt away if I made that foolish decision. As it turns out, Mara announced soon afterward that she'd be moving out of her apartment, and would be relocating to the beach for the summer. hOM Yoga would continue at a yet-to-be-determined location, but, for now, plans to open a studio had been canceled.

Instead, she proposed something else.

"Maybe you'd like to start teaching," Mara said.

"I don't know if I'm qualified," I said.

"I was thinking something like Let's Talk Yoga with Neal."

"But I don't know anything."

"You know enough."

Maybe, she said, there could be a little wine involved, and then an informal discussion of yoga philosophy. These things were usually quite dull, but I could bring an entertaining perspective.

Now I began to get excited.

"OK," I said. "But there has to be some *asana* involved. To loosen the mind. Like a half an hour."

"Do you want me to lead it?" she asked.

"I can handle a half hour," I said. "Can I bring my vaporizer?"

"Hah, hah, vaporizer," said Mara.

"But I'm serious."

"No marijuana, Neal."

Oh, but *wine* was OK. Fine, then. I'd do it without weed.

Just like that, I'd decided to become a yoga teacher. Let's Talk Yoga with Neal, though, would be the worst name for a yoga class since *Lilias, Yoga, and You*. Instead, I decided, the class would be called Club Sutra. That sounded sufficiently fun and pretentious.

With Mara's apartment no longer in play, I had to find an appropriate location for my class. Someone invited me to check out a place called the Against the Stream Buddhist Meditation Society, located on a retail strip of Melrose dominated by anarchist bike shops, art galleries, and a fabulous ice cream shop owned by a mad Japanese chef, whose signature flavors, Brown Bread and Bacon Caramel, ranked among the best scoops I'd ever eaten. The ice cream alone was enough to make me consider Against the Stream as the home for my class.

I also liked the space itself, with its cool finished concrete floors, stark white walls, high-ceilings, and collection of lovely gold Buddha statues. It felt welcoming, unassuming, and calm. On a Sunday morning, I went to Against the Stream for a sit, led by a Buddhist monk wearing a chocolate-brown robe. We meditated quietly for a while, and then he talked about the history of Buddhism and meditation. I found what he had to say very interesting, though I don't remember any of it right now, and I didn't take any notes.

Regardless, I returned a week and a half later for a meditation with the founder of Against the Stream, Noah Levine. On Sunday, there had been maybe fifteen people in the room, but this time it was packed with people, many of them heavily tattooed, though none of them as heavily as Levine himself, who sat calmly on a cushion on a raised platform. The room had more than a faint whiff of AA meetings about it, which made sense. Levine is the author of *Dharma Punx*, a memoir where he details his journey from smoking marijuana for the first time at age six, to a padded detox jail cell eleven years later. His father, Stephen Levine, was a well-known Buddhist author, and when Noah hit bottom, he thought, "Maybe I will try dad's hippie meditation bullshit."

"We all sort of have a different doorway to *dharma* or spiritual practice," he writes in *Dharma Punx*. "Suffering is a doorway. For me it was the suffering of addiction, violence and crime which opened me at a young age, seventeen years old."

When *I* was seventeen, on the other hand, I spent my time going to student-council meetings and padding my résumé for college. While Levine immersed himself in the Southern California punk scene, I worshipped Michael J. Fox in *Family Ties*. My doorway to *dharma* didn't open until the *New York Times* called me fat. I sat there with the other Dharma Punx while Levine led us through a "loving kindness" meditation. This involved him giving us a mantra, and it also involved him talking throughout the entire sit. But I was still figuring out the silent, mantraless meditation. He spoke to me not, at least not that night.

Still, I loved his space, and wanted to use it to teach

my own special brand of yoga nonsense. Renting it proved no problem. I booked the last Tuesday in July and the first Tuesday in August, and, soon after, sent out an email headlined "Neal Pollack Yoga Class." It read:

> Well, I bet you never thought you'd see that in an email subject line, but here we go. I'm teaching my first yoga classes very soon. Please don't be afraid. I've been training for quite some time now, and am working with my trusted teacher, Mara, to develop a fun and interesting program. So here are the particulars:
>
> Hom Yoga Presents
> Neal Pollack's Club Sutra
> Tuesday, July 28 and
> Tuesday, August 4
> 7–9 PM
> @Against the Stream Buddhist Meditation Society
> 4300 Melrose Avenue (between Vermont and the 101)
> Los Angeles
> $10 suggested donation.
>
> You can find more details about what the class will entail on my website.
>
> Classes are available to people at all levels, from absolute beginner to transcendent yoga genius. Enlightenment not guaranteed, but maybe afterward, we'll go across the street for ice cream.
>
> I hope to see you there. Please forward this to anyone you know who might be interested.
>
> Namaste,
> Neal

Almost immediately, my friend Jerod wrote back: "Did you really just send an email to everyone you know asking for $10 so you can teach them yoga? Just checking."

Yes, I thought. *I guess I did.* When I'd started practicing yoga seven years before at the Lance Armstrong 24-Hour Fitness in Northeast Austin, I had stick arms, a donut belly, and a really bad attitude. I definitely didn't think I'd end up teaching other people. Yet in a few weeks, I was going to teach my first yoga class. And I was doing it on purpose.

We visited Regina's family in Nashville for the Fourth of July. At a barbecue, a buddy who I hadn't seen for a while said, "So why, exactly, are you doing this?"

Without thinking for a second, I said, "It's a calling."

"Damn, man," he said. "That sounds religious."

"Yeah," I said. "I guess it does. Well, yoga isn't exactly tied to any one religion, but . . ."

I then proceeded to bore the shit out of him for five minutes.

Sure, I was a little drunk, and more than a little stoned, when I said that yoga was my calling. But even now, though I am, again, a little drunk and more than a little stoned, I still stand by the word. I was humbled by everything my body could do, and even more humbled by everything it couldn't. I saw the world more clearly than ever before. Admittedly, that wasn't very clear at all, but occasionally, surprisingly, there was an open spot in the fog.

I asked Elijah if I should be nervous about teaching my first class.

"Maybe a little," he said, "but no more than that."

That was wise advice from a booger-eater. Still, my

nerves continued, and I looked for encouragement from my yoga colleagues.

"Fake it 'till you make it," said one of them.

All right then, I would.

I spent a few weeks observing Patty's Friday-morning class at Karuna Yoga. She pointed things out to me, and I nodded, trying to show that I understood. On the fourth week, she allowed me to make some adjustments. I told one guy to spread his fingers during downward dog, opened up a couple of people during warrior two, and kindly demonstrated, to a stray beginner, the proper way to put your hands at your heart. Then Patty had the class do handstand. A woman called me over to help. I stood behind her, which you are *not* supposed to do when assisting handstand. You stand in front, so you can catch people when they go up; instead, I failed to catch her on the way down, and she nearly cracked her kneecaps.

"Should I have my head on the wall?" she asked.

"Um, probably not," I said.

After class, I said to Patty, "maybe I shouldn't teach poses that I don't know how to do myself."

"That's wise," she said.

Then came the Monday before my first class. I groaned through yet another horrific Morning Mysore session. Mara had rented out a not-very-clean dance studio on Hyperion so she could continue to wring all the *samskara* out of us. As I wrenched myself toward the end of my practice, I saw Mara and Patty standing a few feet away, looking at me and whispering seriously to each other.

Oh, man, I thought. *I'm in trouble.*

When I was done, Mara squatted beside me and looked at me thoughtfully.

"So I was thinking . . ." she said.

"Oh, crap," I said.

"There are a million people who can teach *asana* better than you."

"Not a *million*," I said.

"Close enough," she said. "But there's no one who can lead a humorous yoga discussion better than you."

"So . . ."

"So I don't think you should teach *asana*. Play to your strengths."

This wasn't bad advice, but I'd spent a lot of time putting together an *asana* program for my class. I didn't have any difficult poses planned, particularly, but it would be about forty minutes, plus another fifteen at the end, designed to calm the mind and keep people receptive to whatever "message" I pulled out of my ass that day. I'd even chosen an awesome soundtrack: Opium Jukebox's hilarious and awesome *bhangra* version of the Sex Pistols album, which should be required listening for all yoga hipsters. Taking out the *asana* left a big hole in my plans. Two hours of "humorous yoga discussion" seemed like a hell of a lot.

Mara was co-sponsoring this event with me, and since she'd sent out emails to her people encouraging them to come bask in my wacky goodness while definitely not emphasizing my *asana* skills. Since she was my teacher, I meekly bowed my consent. I went home and sadly began editing my program.

For some reason, not being allowed to teach *asana* depressed me. I might be able to hold a room for two hours with funny talking. To do it while *exercising*, though, would be a fresh challenge. But it wasn't going to happen. As I adjusted to my new reality and tried to pull together a two-hour talking program, I began to lose all courage, in myself, in my practice, in my work, and in the entire world. Dark ego-drenched clouds of misery and self-doubt hung above me.

"I'm a yoga loser," I sighed. "*Soy un perdedor.*" And then I sighed even deeper, because that reference was now almost twenty years old.

The next morning, I got an email from Mara. She'd been talking to her boyfriend, she wrote, "and he's bummed that I kinda burst the *asana* bubble, because he really wanted to do some yoga with you. Mind you, he's never come to my class! But as you anticipated, this is just the type of guy YOU can bring to yoga—not because you're an expert *asana* instructor, but because you are you. So I'd like to withdraw my remarks from yesterday. Bottom line: you need to teach whatever is in your heart. AND it's going to be a small supportive group tonight, so no matter what you do, we'll love you."

The spirit of yoga goodness had once again lifted me up from despair. Of course, that meant I had to spend all fucking day putting my program back together again. I hadn't even charged my iPod! But Mara had showed me once again why she was my teacher, and I wrote her back in appreciation.

"Dammit, woman," I said. "Make up your mind!"

All day, I paced the house, gnawing on my fingers and murmuring "I'm going to fail, I'm going to fail, I'm going to fail."

"Jesus, Pollack," Regina said. "Detach."

"HOW CAN I DETACH WHEN I'M GOING TO FAIL?" I shouted.

"You're not going to fail."

"NO ONE'S GOING TO COME!"

"Who *cares* if no one comes?"

She had a point, and I stopped hating myself. But I did continue to fill the house with nervous energy. An hour-and-a-half before class, as I straightened a pile of papers on the stairs, Regina said to me, "Just fucking go already!"

From the living room, where he was watching cartoon dogs blow each other up, Elijah yelled, "Teach a good yoga class, daddy!" That line would go direct to video, but the sentiment made my heart warm.

I got to the venue more than an hour early; I drank water, drank tea, went to pee twice, perused the Buddhist literature lending library, and paged through a book of yoga poses on the off chance that I might learn how to teach them in the waning minutes before my first class began. Then I went to my mat and pushed up into headstand. It felt like I held on there for twenty minutes, though realistically, it was probably more like two. Regardless, my head felt clear and ready.

We'd do poses, and a little breath control, maybe sit quietly for a few minutes, and then I'd talk for a while, with no authority at all, about the history and philosophy of yoga. The rest of the time, hopefully to everyone's satisfaction, I'll ramble through pop-cultural digressions and make fart jokes. And, at the end, we'll take some inversions and have a nice *savasana*. If we chanted a little in Sanskrit as well, that was nothing to fear. It would be just like Hebrew School, only more pretentious and half-naked.

By 7 PM, my students had entered: Mara and her boyfriend; Patty; another teacher from Karuna who'd become a good friend; and two of my former fellow *sevas*. It almost felt like a dress rehearsal. The following week, I'd have a dozen students, several of whom I'd never actually met before. That would be a real yoga class. This, on the other hand, just felt like doing yoga with my friends and mentors. If I wanted anything more than that out of life, then I was wanting too much. In the present moment, I felt pure contentment.

I clapped my hands together.

"All right, everyone," I said. "Let's get started."

ALSO BY NEAL POLLACK

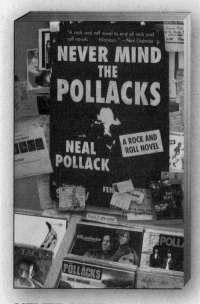

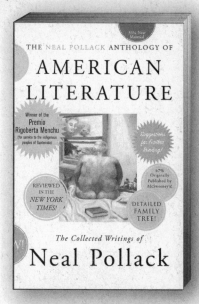

NEVER MIND THE POLLACKS
A Rock and Roll Novel

ISBN 978-0-06-052791-4 (paperback)

The life story of the book's main character, "Neal Pollack," is uniquely American. The only son of Jewish immigrant parents, he shows an aptitude early in life for rock criticism. Prodded by the legendary Sam Phillips, haunted by a ghostly, mysterious blues man, and deeply disturbed by his mother's illegitimate marriage to Jerry Lee Lewis, he leaves his Memphis boyhood behind to become a folk troubadour in Greenwich Village. Six broken hearts, two liver transplants, and a lot of cocaine orgies later, he meets his destiny in a surprise ending that will shock anyone who wasn't paying attention to the early chapters.

"Pollack is a virtuoso."
　　　　　　　—Washington Post Book World

THE NEAL POLLACK ANTHOLOGY OF AMERICAN LITERATURE
The Collected Writings of Neal Pollack

ISBN 978-0-06-000453-8 (paperback)

A collection of satirical pieces including excerpts from Pollack's most popular novels, such as *Leon: A Man of the Streets*, and his most significant non-fiction works, such as his landmark essay on U.S. foreign policy, "The Decision to Invade New Zealand and How It Wasn't Made." Pollack is the author of more than forty books of fiction, non-fiction, poetry, literary criticism, and military history, as well as a winner of several major book awards. Incredibly, this is the first comprehensive collection of his work ever published.

"[A great] satire of authorial vanity."
　　　　　　　—Rolling Stone